40-00

D1380608

Clinics in Developmental Medicine No. 150
CONGENITAL HEMIPLEGIA

© 2000 Mac Keith Press
High Holborn House, 52–54 High Holborn, London WC1V 6RL

Senior Editor: Martin C.O. Bax
Editor: Hilary M. Hart
Managing Editor: Michael Pountney
Sub Editor: Claire Montell

Set in Times and Avant Garde on QuarkXPress

The views and opinions expressed herein are those of the authors and do not necessarily
represent those of the publisher

Accuracy of referencing is the responsibility of the authors

618.928 NEV

First published in this edition 2000

British Library Cataloguing-in-Publication data:
A catalogue record for this book is available from the British Library

POMM

ISSN: 0069 4835
ISBN: 1 898 683 19 0

Printed by The Lavenham Press Ltd, Water Street, Lavenham, Suffolk
Mac Keith Press is supported by Scope (formerly The Spastics Society)

Clinics in Developmental Medicine No. 150

Congenital
Hemiplegia

Edited by

BRIAN NEVILLE
Institute of Child Health, University College London,
Great Ormond Street Hospital for Children NHS
Trust
London, UK

ROBERT GOODMAN
Institute of Psychiatry, King's College London,
South London and Maudsley NHS Trust,
London, UK

2000
Mac Keith Press

Distributed by 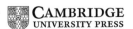 **CAMBRIDGE**
UNIVERSITY PRESS

CONTENTS

AUTHORS' APPOINTMENTS

Jean Aicardi — Honorary Professor, Great Ormond Street Hospital for Children NHS Trust, London, England, UK

Sarah E Aylett — Consultant Paediatric Neurologist, Great Ormond Street Hospital for Children NHS Trust, London, England, UK

J Helen Cross — Consultant Paediatric Neurologist, Great Ormond Street Hospital for Children NHS Trust, London, England, UK

J Keith Brown — Consultant Paediatric Neurologist, Edinburgh Sick Children's NHS Trust, Royal Hospital for Sick Children, Sciennes Road, Edinburgh, Scotland, UK

Roy B Davis — Co-director, Motion Analysis Laboratory, Shriners Hospitals for Children, Greenville, SC, USA

Peter A DeLuca — Orthopaedist, Consultant, Center for Motion Analysis, Connecticut Children's Medical Center, Hartford, CT, USA

Robert Goodman — Professor of Brain and Behavioural Medicine, Institute of Psychiatry, King's College London, South London and Maudsley NHS Trust, De Crespigny Park, Denmark Hill, London SE5 8AF, England, UK

Bengt Hagberg — Professor of Paediatrics (Emeritus), Consultant Child Neurologist, Department of Paediatrics, Göteborg University, The Queen Silvia Children's Hospital, Göteborg, Sweden

Gudrun Hagberg

Consultant Neuropaediatric Epidemiologist, Department of Pediatrics, Göteborg University, The Queen Silvia Children's Hospital, Göteborg, Sweden

Brian Harding

Consultant Neuropathologist, Great Ormond Street Hospital for Children NHS Trust, London, England, UK

Valerie Muter

Honorary Clinical and Research Psychologist, Institute of Child Health, University College London *and* Great Ormond Street Hospital for Children NHS Trust, London, England, UK

Brian Neville

Professor of Paediatric Neurology, Institute of Child Health, University College London WC1N 1EH *and* Great Ormond Street Hospital for Children NHS Trust, London, England, UK

Gerhard Niemann

Consultant Paediatric Neurologist, University Hospital of Tübingen, Department of Child Neurology, Hoppe-Seyler Strasse, Tübingen, Germany

Tom F Novacheck

Pediatric Orthopaedic Associate, Gillette Children's Specialty Healthcare, St Paul *and* Director, Motion Analysis Laboratory, Gillette Children's Specialty Healthcare, St Paul, MN *and* Assistant Professor, Department of Orthopaedic Surgery, University of Minnesota Hospitals, MN, USA

Sylvia Õunpuu

Kinesiologist, Director, Center for Motion Analysis, Connecticut Children's Medical Center, Hartford, CT, USA

David Scrutton

Honorary Senior Lecturer, Institute of Child Health, University College London, London, England, UK

David C Taylor

Honorary Professor of Child and Adolescent Neuropsychiatry, Institute of Child Health, University College London *and* Great Ormond Street Hospital for Children NHS Trust, London.

Paul Uvebrant

Assistant Professor, Department of Paediatric Neurology, The Queen Sylvia Children's Hospital, Göteborg, Sweden

Faraneh Vargha-Khadem

Professor of Developmental Cognitive Neuroscience, Institute of Child Health, University College London, *and* Great Ormond Street Hospital for Children NHS Trust, London, England, UK

E Geoffrey Walsh

Honorary Fellow, Department of Biomedical Science (Physiology), University of Edinburgh, George Square, Edinburgh, Scotland, UK

Lars-Martin Wiklund

Paediatric Neuroradiologist, The Queen Silvia Children's Hospital, Göteborg, Sweden

Carol Yude

Research Psychologist, Institute of Psychiatry, King's College London *and* Chair, HemiHelp, London, England, UK

FOREWORD

How odd a quirk of medical nosology it is to fixate upon a term like 'Congenital Hemiplegia'. Was it, at the time these conditions were named, simply a question of naming the 'cerebral' palsies by their most obvious visible components? Was it because the condition of these infants is defined before the broader implications of the brain disorder have expressed themselves, or could express themselves? Or is it perhaps, because somehow, any reference to the brain disorder seems pejorative? Taxonomy matters because what we call things determines much about how we think about them.

For example, calling this common (5/10 000), cerebral injury 'hemiplegia' might be at the root of the irksomely frequent delay in diagnosis. Front line practitioners might reasonably expect that that is what they should look for when parents start to tell them things are not right. In an important way, the task of this book is to unthink the consequences of the original categorisation. Medical taxonomies usually prove to be overinclusive but it is hard to break old habits of thought even in the light of that knowledge. As this book amply demonstrates, the radiologists, the pathologists, the psychologists and indeed the clinicians themselves have knowledge enough to construct a better taxonomy. A better conceived taxonomy could help make the various outcomes more predictable.

Prediction has a large part to play in medicine; no rational intervention is possible unless we know, in each particular case, what is likely to happen otherwise. A little while ago, I received a tiny box of wedding cake. It was the only communication I had had for 20 years from a family who now wanted me to celebrate with them that outcome of treatment for congenital hemiplegia. I was very touched. All I had done was to address the balance of cost and benefit between the 'security' offered by giving anticonvulsants and the hyperkinesis resulting from taking them. How was I to know, rather than hope, that it would turn out well in the end? Then again, in the early 1970s, I was following up the children with epilepsy in paediatric neurologist turned psychiatrist Kit Ounsted's 1948 series. I visited one patient from his series, a girl on whom the great Hugh Cairns had performed a hemispherectomy in 1950 shortly after Krynauw's report. She was a gentle lady living a comfortable life in elegant surroundings free of many of the distresses that punctuated the lives of others I met with the same congenital disorder. Although one measure of their outcome of the treatment of these two people is the happy contrast with what would otherwise have been likely, there is another, less happy, contrast to be made with what their families had hoped for them at their conception. What might prevent the original misfortunes of the hemispheric abnormality? Knowing that, it seems from this book, is yet a great way off. The prevention and mitigation of the subsequent misfortunes is the business of the various clinicians whose many and diverse activities are included in this volume. Appropriate attention to the wide implications of the cerebral injury can be combined with rational attention to the disordered limb functioning. The book is an excellent clinical manual.

There is also ample material here for considerations that are more academic. Most of the enigmas of developmental neuropsychiatry are here. Why are the sexes unequally represented and in which sorts of condition are they equal? Why, given that it seems, according to Goodman, in the introduction to this book, that Fortuna plays so large a role, are there biases towards left-sided cerebral impairment being more probable? 'The Lord God is subtle', wrote Einstein 'But He does not cheat'. Perhaps Fortuna does it for Him, or perhaps we mistake her mischief for His plan. Is it in the nature of the sort of injury that gives rise to epilepsy that it also creates psychiatric and cognitive problems or does the seizure disorder itself have an importantly disturbing effect? It is clear that there is scope for very fine break down within the various causes and locations of cerebral injury before the analyses of their effects are made. Yet, this is still difficult given the finding, in the Hagbergs' chapter for example, that we remain ignorant of cause in up 40% of cases. What is the reason for the counter intuitive finding that, when not scrambled further by seizures, the brain can perform almost as well with half its resources closed down? Actually, everyone agrees that hemicerebral impairment has massive effects, to whit the reorganisation of language in half the cases for one. If it was 'ordinary' to locate language anywhere handy it would be a waste of time to go to all the trouble the normal brain goes to. The measure of the success of that reorganisation might be better if the family's general level of functioning is taken into consideration. The disappointment for a family of IQ 150 to have a child with a score of a mere 100 was made very plain to me by an angry father.

Freud, by his work on infantile cerebral paralysis, made his only original observation that has stood the test of time. The value of Goodman's long-term research project and the initiative of launching a support process for those affected in this prominently similar way are worth celebrating; it best justifies the continued use of the term 'congenital hemiplegia' as a social category. In consequence of leading an initiative in elective surgery, Neville has shown that it has been worth people developing skills in a number of disciplines that are required in support. Thus clinical epidemiology, paediatric neuroscience, radiology and pathology have derived mutual benefit from the increase in knowledge. Many parents will feel the benefit of their health professional having read this book

DAVID C TAYLOR
Abergavenny 2000

INTRODUCTION
AETIOLOGY AND PATHOGENESIS

Robert Goodman

Families and professionals have many questions about congenital hemiplegia. How should the physical disability be assessed and treated? What are the educational, emotional and social consequences? How should services be organised? Most of the chapters in this volume address exactly these sorts of practical questions, with leading experts from around the world providing the best available answers (and also noting how many pressing questions remain unanswered or poorly answered).

Prior to tackling these practical issues related to assessment and treatment, the first four chapters consider the equally important issue of causation. What has happened to the brain in congenital hemiplegia? And why has it happened? Children and parents naturally want answers to these key questions. Knowing more about causation is relevant not only to prevention but also to relieving unnecessary guilt since parents often blame themselves unfairly, and accurate reassurance can bring enormous relief. For example, one mother was convinced that she was to blame for her son's hemiplegia because he had fallen from her arms and hit his head when he was 6 months old – the hemiplegia was first noticed about a month later. She lived with her guilt for 9 years before an MRI scan showed that the hemiplegia was due to a cerebral malformation that clearly dated back to early pregnancy – it is very typical that the motor disability in congenital hemiplegia only made itself apparent in the second half of the first year of life (see chapter 5). Freed from guilt, the mother not only felt better; she was also able to relate more naturally to her son.

Questions about causation fall into two main groups. There are questions about pathogenesis: what went wrong and when? And there are questions about aetiology: why did this happen to this particular child?

Pathogenesis

Answers to the 'what' and 'when' questions about pathogenesis are beginning to emerge, largely thanks to the neuropathology and neuroimaging studies described in more detail in chapters 2, 3 and 4. In brief, there seem to be three main pathogenic processes, each associated with a different developmental stage: cerebral malformations originating in early fetal life; periventricular lesions largely arising at a gestational age of between 24 and 34 weeks (whether in utero, or after a preterm birth); and cortical infarctions occurring just before or around the time of a term birth. Of course, this three-way classification is a simplification. For example, the group with periventricular lesions can be subdivided on the basis of their MRI appearance according to whether the periventricular damage probably resulted from haemorrhagic infarction or leukomalacia. To complicate matters further, there are also mixed forms and intermediate forms, as well as children with different pathologies or no identifiable pathology at all.

Aetiology
The 'why' question is about aetiology, and there are fewer answers in this domain. The aim of aetiological studies is to identify which genes and environmental risk factors render a fetus liable to congenital hemiplegia. There is no a priori reason to assume that the same genetic and environmental risk factors apply to all the relevant pathogenic processes, e.g. that the risk factors for maldevelopment will be the same as the risk factors for cortical infarction. Studies to date have implicated both genetic and environmental risk factors in at least some individuals. On the genetic side, there are reports of families in which congenital hemiplegia appears to be inherited as an autosomal dominant trait with partial but high penetrance (Haar and Dyken 1977, Berg et al. 1983, Zonana et al. 1986). On the environmental side, as described in chapter 1, preterm birth is a well-recognised risk factor for hemiplegia, even though prematurity is not as strongly associated with hemiplegia as it is with the bilateral spastic cerebral palsies. As also described in chapter 1, there is evidence that hemiplegia is commoner too among term babies who were small for gestational age, and among term and moderately preterm babies whose mothers experienced health problems in pregnancy. But knowing that genes and environment can both influence which children become hemiplegic is not enough; it is also important to establish how powerful these factors are. How fully do genetic and environmental risk factors explain which children develop hemiplegia? Genes and environment are powerful explanatory factors for phenylketonuria or organic mercury poisoning, with important implications for prevention. Is the same true for congenital hemiplegia, or does chance play a much larger role? Unfortunately, studies of the twins and other relatives of individuals with congenital hemiplegia do suggest that chance plays a dominant role – making prevention seem far less feasible.

TWIN STUDIES
Twins are around three times commoner than expected in representative samples of children with congenital hemiplegia. This overrepresentation can largely be explained by the higher rate of preterm birth among twins, though twin-specific risk factors, including the consequences of a co-twin's death in utero, may also play some part (Goodman and Alberman 1996). The most striking finding from twin studies is the lack of concordance for hemiplegia. Combining information from three studies that have looked at twins and triplets with congenital hemiplegia (Griffiths 1967, Petterson et al. 1993, Goodman and Alberman 1996), 59 co-twins were identified who survived for long enough to have manifested the signs of congenital hemiplegia if present; the ratio of monozygotic to dizygotic twins was roughly as expected, and none of the co-twins had hemiplegia or any other form of cerebral palsy (CP). No doubt some concordant twin pairs exist, but it seems safe to conclude that they are relatively rare. This being the case, the heritability of congenital hemiplegia must be low, at least in

twins. Similarly, the lack of concordance argues against a major role for shared environmental factors such as exposure to maternal illness, since these shared factors would presumably affect both twins in many instances, rather than sparing the co-twin in nearly all cases. Nor is there any evidence that it is birth complications that account for the difference between twins with hemiplegia and their unaffected co-twins. For example, in Goodman and Alberman's (1996) study, twins with hemiplegia were no more likely than their unaffected co-twins to be the lighter or second born of the pair.

OTHER FAMILY STUDIES

Since it is possible that twins are a special case, it is important to look at recurrence rates in relatives other than twins. Goodman and Alberman (1996) found that among 155 full biological siblings of a representative sample of singletons with hemiplegia, there were no cases of congenital hemiplegia and only one case of another form of CP. Similarly, in Gustavson and colleagues' (1969) nation-wide Swedish search for identical syndromes of CP in the same family, no family could be identified with more than one member with congenital hemiplegia. Taken together with the twin studies, these family studies suggest that the aetiology of most cases of congenital hemiplegia is not strongly determined by genetic susceptibility, maternal factors, or any of the other environmental factors that are likely to be shared by family members. This does not rule out major genetic or environmental contributions to a small minority of cases, and neither does it rule out relatively weak genetic or environmental contributions for the majority.

IDENTIFIED RISKS ARE RARE OR WEAK

The gene or genes for dominantly inherited forms of hemiplegia seem to be powerful risk factors, with published pedigrees suggesting high penetrance (Haar and Dyken 1977, Berg et al. 1983, Zonana et al. 1986). At the same time, such genes are only likely to account for a very small proportion of congenital hemiplegia; if it were otherwise, the recurrence rates in family members of epidemiological samples of children with congenital hemiplegia would be substantially higher. By contrast, some of the identified environmental risk factors are relatively common, but these are not very powerful, at least if considered in absolute rather than relative terms. For example, although low birthweight is a relatively common risk factor for congenital hemiplegia, under 1% of low-birthweight children develop congenital hemiplegia (Goodman and Alberman 1996) – a low absolute risk even if it is some 10 to 20 times higher than the risk for a child of normal birthweight.

UNIDENTIFIED ENVIRONMENTAL FACTORS OR CHANCE?

It is possible that congenital hemiplegia is determined by some powerful environmental factor that has yet to be identified, and that is not shared by close relatives (including monozygotic twins). For example, hemiplegia could be the result of the placenta being located in just the wrong part of the uterus; co-twins and other siblings would then generally avoid hemiplegia through having a different placental location. It is at least as plausible, though, that chance is the main factor governing who does and does not develop congenital hemiplegia (Goodman and Alberman 1996). This is not to say that the onset of hemiplegia defies the

3

ordinary laws of causality, just as it is not denying causality to say that the number that comes up on a roulette wheel is decided by chance. In everyday speech, it would make sense to say that congenital hemiplegia was largely governed by chance if the condition commonly resulted from complex chains or combinations of minor variations within the normal range, such that the outcome was unpredictable in practice if not in theory.

How Might Chance Work?

Many of the processes involved in brain development are probabilistic rather than deterministic, so chance may play an important part in normal brain development (Goodman 1994). The outcome of probabilistic development will usually be a normal brain but may sometimes be an abnormal brain as a result of chance alone. If so, maldevelopment of one hemisphere could be due to chance factors with little or no contribution from genetic liability or environmental insults – particularly since the asymmetry of the maldevelopment argues against a predominant role for those genetic and environmental influences that would be expected to affect both hemispheres fairly equally. If unilateral malformations could be due to chance, so too could cerebral infarctions. Blockage of a cerebral artery, perhaps by a placentally derived embolus that has passed through the foramen ovale, might be a random low-frequency event that owed little or nothing to genetic predisposition and environmental adversity.

Prospects for Prevention

If predicting in advance which fetus will sustain the brain damage that results in congenital hemiplegia is currently almost as difficult as predicting who will win a lottery, it is not surprising that there are not any specific preventative measures at present. For families with the rare autosomal dominant form of congenital hemiplegia, specific genetic tests and appropriate counselling may one day be available. There are many good reasons for trying to reduce the incidence of prematurity, fetal growth retardation, maternal ill-health and other obstetric complications, and also for continuing to improve the care of preterm infants; succeeding in these areas may reduce the rate of hemiplegia.

REFERENCES

Berg, R. A., Aleck, K. A., Kaplan, A. M. (1983) Familial porencephaly. *Archives of Neurology,* **40,** 567–569.

Goodman, R. (1994) Brain Development. *In:* Rutter, M., Hay, D. F. (Eds) *Development Through Life: A Handbook for Clinicians.* Oxford: Blackwell Scientific Publications, p.49–78.

— Alberman, E. (1996) A twin study of congenital hemiplegia. *Developmental Medicine and Child Neurology,* **38,** 3–12.

Griffiths, M. (1967) Cerebral palsy in multiple pregnancy. *Developmental Medicine and Child Neurology,* **9,** 713–731.

Gustavson, K. H., Hagberg B., Sanner, G. (1969) Identical syndromes of cerebral palsy in the same family. *Acta Paediatrica Scandinavica,* **58,** 330–340.

Haar, L., Dyken, P. (1977) Hereditary nonprogressive athetotic hemiplegia: a new syndrome. *Neurology,* **27,** 849–854.

Petterson, B., Nelson, K. B., Watson, L., Stanley, F. (1993) Twins, triplets, and cerebral palsy in births in Western Australia in the 1980s. *British Medical Journal,* **307,** 1239–1243.

Zonana, J., Adornato, B. T., Glass, S. T., Webb, M. J. (1986) Familial porencephaly and congenital hemiplegia. *Journal of Pediatrics,* **109,** 671–674.

1
ANTECEDENTS

Gudrun Hagberg and Bengt Hagberg

Hemiplegic cerebral palsy (CP) is the most common CP syndrome among children born at term and second only to diplegia among preterm infants (Hagberg et al. 1996). So-called 'congenital' spastic hemiplegia was long considered to be mainly a perinatal problem, presumed to be due to damage at birth (Ingram 1964). However, for term children with hemiplegia, present-day knowledge strongly supports the notion that the brain lesion most often has an intrauterine origin (Molteni et al. 1987, Niemann et al. 1994). In preterm children with hemiplegic CP, as in those with diplegic CP, the pattern of risk factors seems to be dominated by adverse perinatal, particularly early postpartum, compromise associated with preterm birth in general. Compared with preterm diplegias, an excess of prenatal adverse events has been recorded among preterm hemiplegias (Hagberg and Hagberg 1984, Uvebrant 1988).

This chapter aims to present the epidemiology and antecedents of hemiplegic CP over a period of time when perinatal care developed tremendously and technical advances in the genetic, neurometabolic and neuroimaging fields successively provided us with tools for differential diagnosis and detailed delineation of brain damage. The chapter will concentrate on part of our ongoing CP panorama studies in west Sweden, with data mainly from the birth years 1975 to 1990 when the Medical Birth Registration had started in Sweden and we gained access to gestational-age-specific vital statistics as well as a number of pre- and perinatal data which allowed a more detailed analysis. The series comprises 689 cases, excluding cases of CP with an identifiable postnatal (> 28 days of life) cause, and gives population-based information on epidemiological trends and aetiologic background factors. All children were between 4 and 8 years of age at the final delineation of the CP diagnosis and type of syndrome. Individuals born preterm and at term were analysed separately. That is important since the sites and types of cerebral lesions differ depending on the stage of brain development at the time of brain compromise, largely irrespective of an intra- or extrauterine environment (Hagberg and Hagberg 1993). Differences between hemiplegic CP and bilateral spastic CP (including diplegic, tetraplegic and dyskinetic when combined with spasticity) will be highlighted.

Definitions
CP was defined as "an umbrella term covering a group of non-progressive, but often changing, motor-impairment syndromes secondary to lesions or anomalies of the brain

TABLE 1.1
Distribution of CP by syndrome for birth years
1975–1990

	N	%
Hemiplegia	238	35
Bilateral spastic CP	380	55
Other	71	10
Total	689	100

arising in the early stages of development" (Mutch et al. 1992, p. 549). Hemiplegic CP was defined as a unilateral motor disability. That did not exclude subtle neurological signs on the side contralateral to the hemiplegia where hyperactive reflexes and a positive Babinski sign are well known to occur, as was found in 44% of Uvebrant's series (1988), a series overlapping with ours. Dyskinetic/athetoid movements or postures, mainly occurring in the affected hand, were also accepted, as given in 21% by Uvebrant (1988).

General data
Overall, spastic forms of CP dominate strongly, comprising 85 to 95% of CP. In our series, hemiplegic CP comprised 35%, bilateral spastic CP 55% and simple ataxia and pure dyskinetic CP around 5% each (Table 1.1). The distribution of cases according to gestational age varies between the syndromes (Fig. 1.1). The proportion of hemiplegic CP increases with gestational age – in our series, from 14% of the very preterm group to 28% of the moderately preterm and 44% of the term group. In contrast, the proportion of bilateral spastic CP decreased from 81% of the very preterm group to 41% of the term group.

Long-term trend in prevalence of all types of CP
Overall two quite separate secular trends could be seen in the crude CP prevalence, i.e. including all live births (Fig. 1.2). Between 1954 and 1970, there was a decrease from 2.2 to 1.4 cases of CP per 1000 live births, followed by a break in the downward trend and an increase. The CP prevalence in the most recent period of our study, 1987 to 1990, was 2.4 per 1000 live births, which is higher than in the mid 1950s. The change in CP trend mainly reflected changes in the live-birth prevalence of preterm infants, especially referring to those with spastic/ataxic diplegia (Hagberg et al. 1996). Throughout the study, the preterm and low-birthweight rates in the general population remained almost unchanged with only a modest increase in later years. Throughout the 1950s and 1960s obstetric services were gradually centralised to key county hospitals with good basic neonatal care (Hagberg et al. 1996). Perinatal mortality and CP prevalence showed a parallel decline, indicating an improved outcome among survivors. During the 1970s, intensive neonatal care was introduced and gradually expanded geographically and improved technically. The increase in CP prevalence after 1970 is explained as a logical consequence of decreasing perinatal mortality in parallel with a fairly constant rate of CP among increasing cohorts of survivors (Hagberg

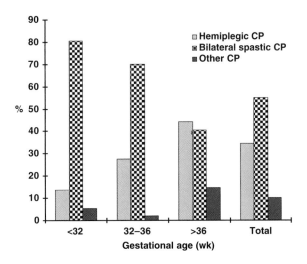

Fig. 1.1 Distribution of hemiplegic CP, bilateral spastic CP and other CP forms by gestational age.

et al. 1982). Identical increasing trends in preterm children have been globally reported, from England, Western Australia, Japan, West Germany, also from the other Nordic countries as previously reviewed (Hagberg et al. 1989).

Long-term trend in prevalence of hemiplegic CP
The trend in the prevalence of preterm hemiplegic CP differed from other forms of preterm CP (see Fig. 1.2). Instead of an initial decrease followed by an increase, the prevalence of hemiplegic CP remained stable over the years. The trend in hemiplegia among babies born at term was very similar to that found for the other forms of term CP, that is a continuous significant slow increase in prevalence.

Trend in the prevalence of gestational-age-specific hemiplegic CP
The gestational-age-specific prevalence of hemiplegia for the birth year period 1975 to 1990 is shown in Figure 1.3. Three gestational age groups were used: the very preterm, the moderately preterm and the term groups. Very preterm birth was considered in the case of birth before 32 completed weeks of gestation; moderately preterm birth between 32 and 36 weeks and term birth after 36 weeks. The very preterm group showed a successive increase in prevalence of hemiplegic CP from 7.1 to 8.3 per 10000 live births. The moderately preterm group showed a marginally decreasing trend and the term group a marginally upward trend. None of these trends were statistically significant, but were in accordance with the corresponding trends of bilateral spastic CP during the same period of time (Krägeloh-Mann et al. 1994). The overall decrease in CP prevalence among moderately preterm infants suggests that progress in intensive care may have led to a decrease in the number of affected children.

7

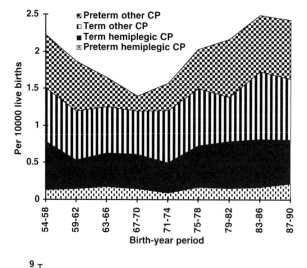

Fig. 1.2 Crude prevalence of CP per 1000 live births between 1954 and 1990.

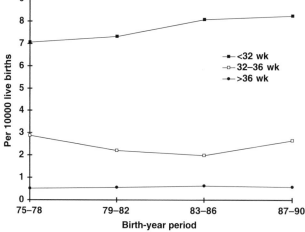

Fig. 1.3 Gestational prevalence of hemiplegic CP between 1975 and 1990.

Antecedents

Preterm birth is a well-established risk factor for CP. The prevalence of CP rises sharply with both lower gestational age and birthweight. This applies above all to bilateral spastic CP and to hemiplegic CP to a lesser degree. In our series, the very preterm infant had a risk of hemiplegic CP 13 times higher than a term infant and of bilateral spastic CP 84 times higher.

The timing of adverse events to the developing brain determines the anatomical localisation and type of lesion and thus the final neurological picture. Ultrasound scans, CT and MRI are of invaluable help nowadays in elucidating sites, extensions, timing and development of lesions (Wiklund et al. 1990, 1991a,b; de Vries et al. 1993; Niemann et al. 1994; Rademaker et al. 1994). Findings of brain maldevelopments point distinctly to an

8

TABLE 1.2.

TABLE 1.2.
Criteria for aetiological classification[a]

Prenatal
    Familial forms with Mendelian inheritance
    Defined prenatal syndromes – chromosomal abnormalities
    Verified congenital infections (toxoplasmosis, rubella, cytomegalovirus, herpes)
    Cerebral maldevelopments, including unspecified prenatal hydrocephalus and unspecified
      microcephaly
    Multiple congenital anomalies/mental retardation (MCA/MR) syndromes
    Intracranial haemorrhage/stroke with confirmed prenatal onset

    For term children
    Indications of periventricular leukomalacia on CT scan in cases with an uneventful delivery and
      neonatal period

Peri/neonatal
    Intracranial haemorrhage/stroke with confirmed peri/neonatal onset. For term children any grade.
      For preterm children only grades III or IV.
    Confirmed brain oedema or concrete evidence of neonatal shock (asystole and need for
      resussitation and organ failure)
    Bacteraemia or CNS infection with confirmed peri/neonatal onset

    For term children
    Hypoxic–ischaemic encephalopathy with at least two of the following symptoms/signs: Apgar
      score <5 at 1 or 5 minutes, resuscitation/ventilation, convulsions before day 3

    For preterm children
    Normal early neonatal ultrasound combined with indications on later CT of periventricular
      leukomalacia and/or periventricular haemorrhage and not meeting the criteria for a prenatal
      aetiology
    Low Apgar scores or low pH (Apgar score <3 at 5 minutes or Apgar score <5 at 10
      minutes, or pH ≤6.9)
    Mechanical ventilation >7 days or complicated by pneumothorax

[a] When overlap between prenatal and peri/neonatal criteria occurred, the following peri/neonatal symptoms/signs took precedence: confirmed appearance of intracranial haemorrhage/stroke, confirmed brain oedema and concrete evidence of neonatal shock. Otherwise prenatal factors had precedence.

early fetal origin on a genetic or clastic basis occurring during the first 20 weeks of brain development. Periventricular pathology such as reduction of periventricular white matter with enlargement of the lateral ventricles is considered to be residual of periventricular leukomalacia/periventricular haemorrhage. These conditions reflect hypo-/hyperperfusion lesions to the immature brain occurring early in the third trimester when the periventricular structures are particularly vulnerable and are considered hazards of the well-recognised fragility of the periventricular watershed areas in the 26th to 34th week of gestation. In contrast, late in the third trimester in the more mature brain, cortical/subcortical structures are more vulnerable and the pathology known to reflect partly major vascular catastrophies, partly hypoxic–ischaemic lesions.

Our criteria for aetiological classification are given in Table 1.2. According to these, each child was allocated to a prenatal, peri-/neonatal, or unclassifiable group. The criteria are practically identical to those used in a recent German–Swedish collaborative study (in

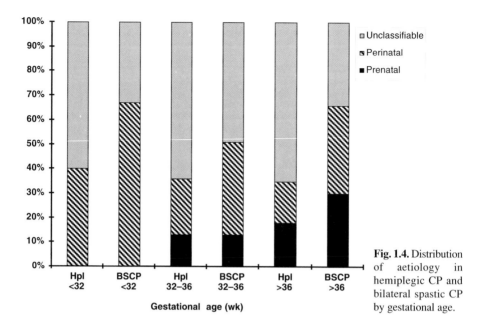

Legend:
- □ Unclassifiable
- ▨ Perinatal
- ■ Prenatal

X-axis labels:
Hpl <32 | BSCP <32 | Hpl 32–36 | BSCP 32–36 | Hpl >36 | BSCP >36

Gestational age (wk)

Fig. 1.4. Distribution of aetiology in hemiplegic CP and bilateral spastic CP by gestational age.

Tübingen, Germany and Göteborg, Sweden) on bilateral spastic CP (Krägeloh-Mann et al. 1995). In the Krägeloh-Mann study we used clinical data from well-designed studies which have been shown to have a high probability for association with cerebral damage. In addition to the clinical symptoms/signs, we used findings from early neonatal ultrasound or CT, as well as CT or MRI findings from examinations later during childhood. The aetiological criteria differed somewhat between term and preterm infants. For preterm infants, an early neonatal normal ultrasound investigation with a later CT scan showing signs of periventricular leukomalacia in the form of periventricular atrophy, was taken as evidence of a cerebral insult which had occurred perinatally. In term infants a prenatal aetiology was considered when there were indications of periventricular leukomalacia on CT scan in individuals with an uneventful delivery and neonatal period. For preterm babies, only intracranial haemorrhage grades III (intraventricular with ventricular dilatation) and IV (intraventricular with parenchymal haemorrhage) were considered sufficient for allocation to the perinatal aetiological group. The reason was that intracranial haemorrhage grades I (subependymal) and II (intraventricular) in preterm infants have been reported not to be specifically related to major disability. The hypoxic–ischaemic encephalopathy criterion was not used for preterm children since in this population there is no direct correlation between defective regulation of cerebral blood flow causing ischaemia and the commonly used indicators of perinatal asphyxia, and because seizures after hypoxic–ischaemic insults are more sporadic. Instead we chose to quantify the severity of parameters when a relation to hypoxic–ischaemic events was known. Apgar scores below 3 at 5 minutes or 5 at 10 minutes or a pH below 7, or mechanical ventilation lasting more than 7 days, or when complicated by pneumothorax,

TABLE 1.3

Distribution of aetiology of hemiplegic CP in 51 children born at term in 1987–1990. Cases are classified according to first criterion met in the respective group.

Aetiology	n	(%)
Prenatal		
Cerebral maldevelopment		
Disturbances of migration	2[a]	
Hemiatrophy	1[a]	
Intracranial haemorrhage/stroke with confirmed prenatal onset	3[a]	
Signs of periventricular leukomalacia on CT scan		
with intrauterine hydrocephalus	1	
without clinical criteria	9[a]	
Total	16	(31)
Perinatal		
Intracranial haemorrhage/stroke	4	
Brain oedema/neonatal shock	1	
Sepsis/CNS infection		
Staphylococcus aureus	1	
Beta-streptococcus	1	
Hypoxic–ischaemic encephalopathy	2	
Total	9	(18)
Unclassifiable	26	(51)

[a] Revealed at CT scan.

were considered sufficient peri/neonatal criteria. As a rule, criteria for a prenatal aetiology took, according to our definitions, precedence over peri/neonatal ones. The exceptions were severe neonatal morbidity in the form of confirmed perinatal intracranial haemorrhage, brain oedema and neonatal shock, which were given priority. The reason was well-established clinical experience that these events comprise objective evidence of neonatal brain compromise sufficient to explain a brain insult resulting in hemiplegic CP.

Figure 1.4 gives a summarised comparison between the aetiology of hemiplegic CP and bilateral spastic CP, with our criteria applied. For both unilateral and bilateral spastic CP the proportion of a peri/neonatal aetiology was highest in the very preterm group comprising 40% of hemiplegic and 67% of bilateral spastic CP. The proportion decreased with gestational age and was 17% among term children with hemiplegia and 36% among term children with bilateral spasticity. A prenatal aetiology could not be verified in any single case in the very preterm group. In term children, a prenatal aetiology was considered very likely in 18% of those with hemiplegia and in 30% of those with bilateral spastic CP.

A detailed list of the distribution of CP according to aetiology is given in Tables 1.3 and 1.4 for term and preterm children. As there was a gradually increasing access to brain imaging with time in the study area and thus we got important information complementary to the clinical assessment, we restricted the detailed analysis to the most recent birth years – 1987 to 1990. For children born at term a prenatal aetiology was considered very likely

TABLE 1.4

Distribution of aetiology of hemiplegic CP in 13 children born moderately preterm and 7 children born very preterm between 1987–1990. Cases are classified according to first criterion met in the respective group.

Aetiology	< 32 wk		32–36 wk	
	n	%	n	%
Prenatal				
Congenital infection (cytomegalovirus)	0		1	
Intracranial haemorrhage/stroke with confirmed prenatal onset				
With intrauterine hydrocephalus	0		1	
Without clinical criteria	0		1[a]	
Signs of periventricular leukomalacia (PVL) on CT scan	0		1[a]	
Total	0	(0)	4	(31)
Perinatal				
Intracranial haemorrhage grade III or IV	3		4	
Signs of PVL with normal initial ultrasound	0		1	
Low Apgar score and low pH	1		0	
Total	4	(57)	5	(38)
Unclassifiable	3	(43)	4	(31)

[a] Revealed at CT scan.

in 16 children (31%) and a perinatal in nine (18%). No likely cause could be found in 26 children (52%). The moderately preterm group comprised 13 children. Four children had a very likely prenatal aetiology of hemiplegia, five a perinatal one, and in four children there was no likely evidence of origin. The very preterm group comprised seven children. None of these had any support for a prenatal aetiology, four had a very likely perinatal aetiology and in three the aetiology was unclassifiable.

Brain imaging had not been systematically performed on all our patients. Results from early ultrasound scans were available in all cases where the neonatal period had been compromised. The findings confirmed a peri/neonatal intracranial haemorrhage/stroke in all cases classified as having one. In addition there was one moderately preterm infant with hemiplegia who had a prenatal intracranial haemorrhage revealed. CT scans had been performed in 47 of the 71 cases that is in 66%. Seven of them had also undergone MRI investigations. The CT/MRI findings never contradicted the aetiological conclusions from the clinical assessment. They either confirmed or underlined the clinically based aetiology, or convincingly indicated a time-related pathology which would otherwise have been considered unclassifiable. Thus, in one half of the term children in which CT/MRI had been performed, CT/MRI settled the timing and type of brain lesion. CT/MRI was normal in 15 of the 47 children investigated (32%). Four of these 15 had a clear perinatal aetiology clinically of CP and in the remaining 11 no likely aetiology was found. Had CT/MRI scans been performed on all our patients, periventricular and cortical/subcortical atrophy would

TABLE 1.5
Prenatal risk factors in hemiplegic CP compared to bilateral spastic CP and in control individuals by gestational age group. Hemiplegic CP and bilateral spastic CP refer to birth years 1975–1990, control individuals to birth years 1967–1982 (Uvebrant 1988).

Gestational age (wk)	Failure in previous pregnancies %	Uterine bleeding %	Preeclamptic signs %	Maternal disorder %	Multiple birth %	Small for gestational age %
<32						
Hemiplegic CP ($n=20$)	21.1	42.1	5.0	25.0	20.0	0.0
Bilateral spastic CP ($n=117$)	16.2	36.2	6.0	19.7	21.4	2.6
Control subjects ($n=44$)	9.1	34.1	4.5	9.1	16.8[b]	2.3
32–36						
Hemiplegic CP ($n=39$)	17.9	17.9	7.7	20.5[a]	12.8	7.7
Bilateral spastic CP ($n=99$)	12.8	16.5	11.1	19.2[a]	12.1	11.1
Control subjects ($n=132$)	11.4	28.0	4.5	6.8	13.6[b]	3.8
>36						
Hemiplegic CP ($n=179$)	5.6	8.0	3.9	11.2[a]	2.2	5.6[a]
Bilateral spastic CP ($n=164$)	6.7	7.1	7.9	10.4[a]	1.2	8.5[a]
Control subjects ($n=269$)	3.0	3.7	3.0	5.6	1.3[b]	1.5

Failure in previous pregnancies defined as ≥ 2 spontaneous abortions and/or stillbirth and/or perinatal death.
Preeclamptic signs defined as mild BP ≥ 140 or ≥ 90 + proteinuria, severe BP ≥ 160 or ≥ 110 both at least at two occasions.
Maternal disorder defined as chronic disorder, pyelonephritis, fever >38.5 at delivery etc.
Small for gestational age defined as ≤ -2 SD from the mean on a Swedish growth chart (Niklasson et al. 1991).
[a]p level ≤ 0.05.
[b]Medical Birth Registration, birth years 1980–1990.

probably have been revealed in additional cases, mainly supporting a prenatal aetiology.

In a representative series of 111 children with hemiplegia, CT scans showed maldevelopment in 17%, periventricular atrophy in 42%, cortical/subcortical atrophy in 12%, other findings in 3% and normal findings in 26% (Wiklund et al. 1990). Changes in the white matter can be depicted with greater sensivity using MRI. Niemann and colleagues (1994) investigated a representative series of 41 hemiplegic children with MRI. They found maldevelopment in 7%, periventricular atrophy in 56%, cortical/subcortical atrophy in 10%, other findings in 10% and normal findings in 17%.

Predisposing factors
Although it is now widely accepted that in the large majority of very preterm children with CP the final brain damage – in a chain of pathogenetic adverse events – occurs in the first week of life, a wide variety of prior prenatal predisposing risk factors and pathways may have occurred (Hagberg and Hagberg 1993). Table 1.5 shows the incidence of selected 'traditional' risk factors among children with hemiplegic and bilateral spastic CP related to gestational age groups. All of these predisposing factors have been shown to be associated

with an increased risk of CP (Hagberg and Hagberg 1984, Uvebrant 1988). When compared to a control group of children without CP or infantile hydrocephalus and born between 1967 and 1982 (Uvebrant 1988), the proportion of risk factors in the cases were usually higher than in the control subjects in all the gestational age groups (see Table 1.5). The individual items 'maternal disorder' in the moderately preterm and term groups and 'small for gestational age' in the term group were, however, the only items that were significantly more frequent in individuals with CP compared to control individuals. The item 'maternal disorder' comprised a mishmash of different but clear disturbances in maternal health during the actual pregnancy. The most common disorder among mothers of preterm infants was fever at delivery and among mothers of term babies chronic disorders of different kinds. Recently, the combination of intrauterine infection and premature rupture of membranes has been shown to be associated with a very high risk of periventricular leukomalcia (Zupan et al. 1996, Dammann and Leviton 1997).

Concluding remarks

In their classical neuropathological CP study 30 years ago, Christensen and Melchior (1967) pessimistically stated that "any postmortem study of neuropathology in hemiplegics is bound to be unrepresentative as most of these patients survive for a long time". Nevertheless, the importance of circulatory disturbances during pregnancy for the origin of prenatal encephalopathies in general, and congenital hemiplegias in particular, was postulated early on by Lyon (1961, 1970) and Lyon and Robain (1967) based on combined clinical and neuropathological observations. Additional confirmatory evidence for a prenatal aetiology was then presented by Goutières and coworkers (1972) and was also supported by studies of Michaelis and colleagues (1980), ourselves (Hagberg et al. 1976) and Uvebrant (1988). The present study, in addition, has pinpointed the high frequency of intracranial bleedings of various kinds that occur perinatally not only in very preterm infants but also in the other gestational age groups.

Today, with access to refined neuroimaging techniques, we have sensitive tools to elucidate abnormal brain pathology early in life and thereby better possibilities to trace and understand the underlying pathogenesis. In parallel, modern obstetrics and neonatology has given us more systematised information on pre- and perinatal clinical data and their correlation to the antecedents of the various CP syndromes. To cover population-based, and thus representative series of cases, in all these respects is problematic due to insufficient resources and availability of technical equipment.

With present-day knowledge, the following aetiopathogenetic main groups underlying hemiplegic CP can be summarised.

MALDEVELOPMENTS

This occurs in a small group of 5 to 15% of those with hemiplegic CP. These children were mainly born at term and only exceptionally very preterm. The aetiology is generally revealed first at neuroimaging. The pathology is, according to our and other investigators' experiences (Wiklund et al. 1990, Niemann et al. 1994), practically always migrational abnormalities such as schizencephaly and focal pachygyria, probably mainly originating from brain development early in the second trimester of pregnancy. The basic cause has so far remained unknown. Cases with familial occurrence can be regarded as practically non-existent (Goodman and Alberman 1996). The pre- and perinatal history is generally uncomplicated. There is a preponderance of upper-limb dominance in motor disability.

PERIVENTRICULAR PATHOLOGY

This is the by far largest group comprising around 40 to 50% among both term and preterm children with hemiplegic CP. The major pathogenetic process is considered to refer to hypo/hyperperfusion in the fragile vascular periventricular area, indicated to occur in the 26th to 34th week of brain development, and finally resulting in classical periventricular leukomalacia and atrophy (Wiklund et al. 1991a, b: Niemann et al. 1994). Extremely preterm infants with very early myelin deficiences secondary to germinal matrix destructions could not be delineated with our limited methodology. Among term children, the periventricular leukomalacia is considered to have occurred during intrauterine life and among preterm children mainly postpartum. Among very preterm infants a more complex and partly different periventricular pathology, often asymmetric, predominates. The more marked the immaturity is, the more prominent are the haemorrhagic components in the periventricular lesions, also the atypical forms, and parallel to that the clinical asymmetries in motor disability (Volpe 1989, Niemann et al. 1994). Among term infants, correlates to clinical antecedents are seldom revealed and brain pathology is first found at neuroimaging. Among preterm infants a complicated early neonatal period is common, often including findings of intracranial haemorrhages of grade III or IV. The motor disability is most often leg dominated.

CORTICAL–SUBCORTICAL PATHOLOGY

This is, according to our experience, a group of around 10 to 15% of those with hemiplegic CP. Two-thirds of individuals are born at term and one-third moderately preterm. The pathogenesis is indicated to have been a vascular catastrophy occurring late in the third trimester. The pre- and perinatal history is still generally unrevealing and the brain pathology first found at neuroimaging. Only a minority of cases can be referred to an obvious perinatal compromise. Cortical and subcortical malacia and atrophy found on CT and MRI scans are sometimes impressive in size in relation to a comparatively modest motor disability. Both upper- and lower-limb dominance in motor disability can be found.

UNTRACEABLE AETIOLOGY

This is still a considerable group of around 30 to 40% of individuals with hemiplegic CP. According to our criteria, no obvious clinical antecedents were found and neuroimaging is normal. The majority of these cases refer to term children where the pre- and perinatal history has been completely normal. A somewhat smaller group comprises preterm children with a perinatal history of varying complication, yet without evidence of pathology at CT and/or MRI.

ACKNOWLEDGEMENT

The studies were supported by grants from the foundations of Folke Bernadotte for Children with Cerebral Palsy and the Frimurare-Barnhusdirektionen in Göteborg.

REFERENCES

Christensen, E., Melchior, J. (1967) *Cerebral Palsy. A Clinical and Neuropathological Study. Clinics in Developmental Medicine No. 25.* London: Spastics International Medical Publications.

Dammann, O., Leviton, A. (1997) Maternal intrauterine infection, cytokines, and brain damage in the preterm newborn. *Pediatric Research,* **42,** 1–8.

De Vries, L.S., Eken, P., Groenendaal, F., van Haastert, I.C., Meiners, L.C. (1993) Correlation between the degree of periventricular leucomalacia diagnosed using cranial ultrasound and MRI later in infancy in children with cerebral palsy. *Neuropediatrics,* **24,** 263–268.

Goodman, R., Alberman, E. (1996) A twin study of congenital hemiplegia. *Developmental Medicine and Child Neurology,* **38,** 3–12.

Goutières, F., Challamel, M-J., Aicardi, J., Gilly, R. (1972) Les hémiplégies congénitales. Sémiologie, étiologie et prognostic. *Archive Française Pédiatrie,* **29,** 839–851.

Hagberg, B., Hagberg, G. (1984) Prenatal and perinatal risk factors in a survey of 681 Swedish cases. *In:* Stanley F, Alberman E, (Eds). *The Epidemiology of the Cerebral Palsies. Clinics in Developmental Medicine No. 87.* London: Spastics International Medical Publications. p 116–134.

—— (1993) The origins of cerebral palsy. *In:* David, T.J. (Ed.). *Recent Advances in Paeditrics.* Edinburgh: Churchill Livingstone. p. 67–83.

—— Olow, I. (1976) The changing panorama of cerebral palsy in Sweden 1954-70. III. The importance of fetal deprivation of supply. *Acta Paediatrica Scandinavica,* **65,** 403–408.

—— —— (1982) Gains and hazards of intensive neonatal care: an analysis from Swedish cerebral palsy epidemiology. *Developmental Medicine and Child Neurology,* **24,** 13–19.

—— Zetterström, R. (1989) Decreasing perinatal mortality – increase in cerebral palsy morbidity. *Acta Paediatrica Scandinavica,* **78,** 664–70.

—— Olow, I. (1996) The changing panorama of cerebral palsy in Sweden. VII. Prevalence and origin during the birth year period 1987-90. *Acta Paediatrica,* **85,** 954–960.

Ingram, T.T.S. (1964) *Paediatric Aspects of Cerebral Palsy.* Edinburgh: E & S Livingstone.

Krägeloh-Mann, I., Hagberg, G., Meisner, Ch., Schelp, B., Haas, G., Edebol Eeg-Olofsson, K., Selbmann, H.K., Hagberg, B., Michaelis, R. (1994) Bilateral spastic cerebral palsy – A comparative study between south-west Germany and western Sweden. II. Epidemiology *Developmental Medicine and Child Neurology,* **36,** 473–483.

—— —— Haas, G., Edebol Eeg-Olofsson, K., Selbman, H.K., Hagberg, B., Michaelis, M. (1995) Bilateral spastic cerebral palsy – A collaborative study between southwest Germany and western Sweden. III. Aetiology. *Developmental Medicine and Child Neurology,* **37,** 191–203.

Lyon, G. (1961) First signs and mode of onset of congenital hemiplegia. In: *Hemiplegic Cerebral Palsy in Children and Adults. Little Club Clinics in Developmental Medicine No. 4.* London: National Spastics Society. p 33–38.

— (1970) Les encéphalopathies congénitales non évolutives. *Louvain Médicale,* **89,** 341–353.

— Robain, O. (1967) Encéphalopathies circulatoires prénatales et paranatales. *Acta Neuropathologica,* **9,** 79–98.

Michaelis, R., Rooschuz, B., Dopfer, R. (1980) Prenatal origin of congenital spastic hemiparesis. *Early Human Development,* **4,** 243–255.

Molteni, B., Oleari, G., Fedrizzi, E. (1987) Relation between CT patterns, clinical findings and etiologic factors in children born at term, affected by congenital hemiparesis. *Neuropediatrics,* **18,** 75–80.

Mutch L, Alberman E, Hagberg B, Kodama K, Velickovic M. (1992) Cerebral palsy epidemiology: where are we now and where are we going? *Developmental Medicine and Child Neurology,* **34,** 547–555.

Niemann, G.,Wakat, J-P., Krägeloh-Mann, I., Grodd, W., Michaelis, R. (1994) Congenital hemiparesis and periventricular leukomalacia: pathogenetic aspects on magnetic resonance imaging. *Developmental Medicine and Child Neurology,* **36,** 943–950.

Niklasson, A., Ericson, A., Fryer, J.G., Karlberg, J., Lawrence, C., Karlberg, P. (1991) An update of the Swedish reference standards for weight, length and head circumference at birth given gestational age (1977-1981). *Acta Paediatrica Scandinavica,* **80,** 756–762.

Rademaker, K.J., Groenendaal, F., Jansen, G.H., Eken, P., de Vries, L.S. (1994) Unilateral haemorrhagic parenchymal lesions in the preterm infant: shape site and prognosis. *Acta Paediatrica,* **83,** 602–608.

Uvebrant, P. (1988) Hemiplegic cerebral palsy. Aetiology and outcome. *Acta Paediatrica Scandinavica,* **Suppl. 345,** 1–100.

16

Wiklund, L.-M., Uvebrant, P., Flodmark, O. (1990) Morphology of cerebral lesions in children with congenital hemiplegia. A study with computed tomography. *Neuroradiology, 32,* 179–186.

— Uvebrant, P., Flodmark, O. (1991a) Computed tomography as an adjunct in etiological analysis of hemiplegic cerebral palsy. I: children born preterm. *Neuropediatrics, 22,* 50–56.

— — — (1991b) Computed tomography as an adjunct in etiological analysis of hemiplegic cerebral palsy. II: children born at term. *Neuropediatrics, 22,* 121–128.

Volpe, J.J. (1989) Current concepts of brain injury in the premature infant. *American Journal of Radiology, 153,* 243–251.

Zupan, V., Gonzales, P., Lacaze-Masmonteil, T., Boithias, C., dÁllest, A.-M., Dehan, M., Gabilan, J.-C. (1996) Periventricular leucomalacia: risk factors revisited. *Developmental Medicine and Child Neurology, 38,* 1061–1067.

2
NEUROPATHOLOGY

Brian Harding

To the morphologist the plethora of lesions encountered in children with hemiplegia is a microcosm of pediatric neuropathology. Prenatal destructive and malforming conditions, the structural consequences of perinatal hypoxia–ischemia, and a variety of postnatally acquired vascular, inflammatory and epileptic disorders all contribute in varying degree to the polymorphic pathology of cerebral palsy in general and childhood hemiplegia in particular. Different pathological changes may produce similar semiology thus undermining the utility of a morphological classification for childhood hemiplegia. Conversely, aetiological classifications have proved impracticable, given the diverse consequences of, for example, intrauterine vascular compromise or birth asphyxia. The purpose of this chapter will, therefore, be less ambitious, cataloguing rather than classifying the wide spectrum of abnormalities, while recognising that this account may be skewed towards the more severe end of the clinical spectrum where morbidity or mortality more usually make biopsy or autopsy material available for pathological study.

Malformations

Cerebral malformations form a small but distinct cohort of childhood hemiplegias. They may be loosely described as neuronal migration defects (Harding et al. 1997, Ellison et al. 1998), by which it is assumed that interference with neuroblast migration in the developing cerebral mantle leads to disturbance in both cortical structure and cellular differentiation. Although diverse in form and anatomical extent, in the clinical context of hemiplegia most of one hemisphere is usually involved, and the resultant lateralised seizures frequently bring these patients to surgical and subsequent neuropathological attention. Three principal types are considered below, and although usually distinct they can occasionally be combined.

Agyria/Pachygyria

These terms refer respectively to absent gyration, or reduced numbers of broadened convolutions (Fig. 2.1), but this is only part of the story. An accurate definition requires microscopic recognition of an abnormally thickened and layered cortical ribbon ('pachy' is after all the Greek for thick); it is a mistake just to equate a smooth surface only with pachygyria. Both radiologists and pathologists have a tendency to use either the terms agyria or lissencephaly rather imprecisely for the macroscopic description of a smooth surface, and macrogyria or pachygyria for coarse widened convolutions. However, a smooth surface may overlie not only

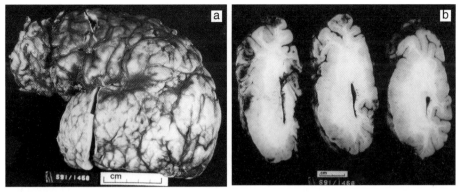

Fig. 2.1. *(a)* Lateral aspect of a surgical hemispherectomy specimen showing the almost completely smooth surface of pachygyria. *(b)* Coronal slices of the specimen shown in fig. 1a. There are hardly any gyral indentations and the cortical ribbon over the lateral aspect is 3 times the normal thickness. For comparison note the normal thickness of the calcarine cortex on the mesial aspect of the occipital lobe.

histologic pachygyria (lissencephaly type I) but also cerebroocular dysplasia (lissencephaly type II), polymicrogyria, or other forms of cortical dysplasia. The characteristic histologic appearance of pachygyria is a thickened cortex of four layers: molecular layer, thin external neuronal layer, sparsely cellular layer including a tangential myelin layer, and finally a very thick inner nerve-cell zone which may fragment into columns interdigitated by narrow bands of radial myelinated fibres. But many variations are possible and layering may be almost imperceptible. In addition nodules of ectopic grey matter regularly occur either within the underlying rather reduced white matter or in the subependymal zone. Rarely pachygyria is combined with polymicrogyria. Considerations of cortical anatomy and the association of olivary heterotopia in the severest bilateral forms sets the pathogenetic determination time for pachygyria towards the end of the first trimester, but the condition is sporadic in its hemiplegic form.

Polymicrogyria
The essence of polymicrogyria is histological. Its appearance to the naked eye is often misleading: the basic gyral pattern can be retained, but the surface may look smooth like pachygyria or roughened akin to cobblestones. Histologically the polymicrogyric cortex is thinner than normal, the miniature convolutions excessively folded and fused giving a map-like configuration in section. Another common feature is the cell-poor molecular layer reaching down perpendicularly into the cortical ribbon in a branched finger-like pattern. This is particularly the case in the unlayered form of polymicrogyria, by far the most commonly encountered in my experience. Rarer is the four-layered subtype in which a cell-poor layer divides the cellular zone into two bands. Other associated features of aberrant neuronal migration include leptomeningeal glioneuronal heterotopia and nodular heterotopia in the white matter, and even pachygyria rarely. The degree of the polymicrogyric malformation is extremely varied. It can extend diffusely through one or both cerebral hemispheres, or be bilateral and symmetric in a particular arterial territory, usually middle

cerebral; but the degree of involvement of the hemispheres may be markedly asymmetrical. It may surround porencephalic or hydranencephalic defects, or may be restricted to the opercular region or the depths of the insula, and it can also be focal. Cingulate and striate cortex are never affected. As a further complication, unilateral involvement may result in either an asymmetrically larger (Fig. 2.2) or smaller (Fig 2.3) hemisphere, all of which are important considerations when trying to correlate pathology with clinical signs of hemiplegia in a patient whose neuroimaging demonstrates hemimegalencephaly. Patho-aetiogenesis is very varied, but most examples are sporadic and consequent upon intrauterine hypoxic–ischaemic insult in the middle trimester, including the perfusional disorders of twinning. Rarer causes include intrauterine infection, certain metabolic disorders including Pelizaeus–Merzbacher disease, glutaric aciduria type II, maple syrup urine disease, peroxisomal disorders and mitochondrial respiratory chain deficiency, and finally polymicrogyria occurs in X-linked Aicardi syndrome and a few autosomal recessive cases. The two principal pathogenetic theories for polymicrogyria invoke either an interference with neuronal migration or a postmigrational midpallial necrosis. Clinical observations, experimental manipulations and cytoarchitectonic studies in polymicrogyria give divergent opinions regarding the determination time of polymicrogyria: from 12 weeks' gestation to as late as 24 weeks'.

Cortical dysplasia with cytomegaly in hemimegalencephaly
This intriguing lesion was first reported by Taylor and colleagues (1971) in surgical specimens from patients treated for focal epilepsy. But the same mixture of abnormal cortical organisation and cytological atypia also occurs in tuberous sclerosis and in a particular and increasingly observed form of hemimegalencephaly (Fig. 2.4) responsible for medically intractable seizures and hemiplegia. Very large, possibly deafferented polyploid neurones with irregular dendritic trees and dispersed Nissl substance, usually demonstrating up-regulation of neurofilament proteins with immunohistochemistry and tangle formation with silver impregnation, are scattered haphazardly across a widened but relatively cell-depleted cortex, or are arranged in clusters or columns. Normal gyrification and lamination are absent, the surface may be smooth or have small sulci, the cell layer may undulate or separate into four layers. The border between grey and white matter is blurred. Varying degrees of astrocytic dysplasia are also encountered. Balloon cells, though much discussed because of their controversial cytogenesis, may be frequent or not evident. Appearances suggest they are atypical astrocytes, but they may not express glial fibrillary acidic protein

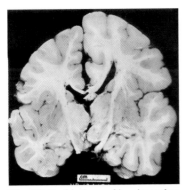

Fig. 2.2. In this form of hemimegalencephaly the abnormal larger hemisphere exhibits extensive polymicrogyria of the frontal, insular and superior temporal cortex.

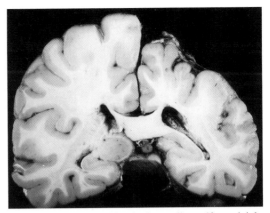

Fig. 2.3. The cortical ribbon in the smaller malformed right hemisphere is irregularly thickened by the miniature but fused gyri of polymicrogyria.

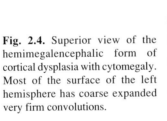

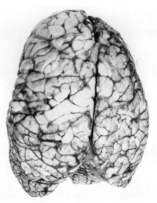

Fig. 2.4. Superior view of the hemimegalencephalic form of cortical dysplasia with cytomegaly. Most of the surface of the left hemisphere has coarse expanded very firm convolutions.

(GFAP), the hallmark of differentiated astrocytes, or on the contrary colocalise it with vimentin or synaptophysin, a neuronal marker (Duong et al. 1994). Astrocytic involvement may be massive on occasion mimicking a tumour, and can extend deeply into the subcortical white matter along with atypical neurones. Sometimes cystic rarefaction or extravagant Rosenthal fibre formation can trap the unwary into a diagnosis of Alexander disease. The hemimegalencephalic form is strictly unilateral.

Hypoxic–ischemic lesions
Reference to Table 2.1 gives some indication of the great variety of structural manifestations attendant upon major embarrassments of cerebral perfusion or oxygen delivery to the developing brain whatever their ultimate causation (Rorke et al. 1992, Harding et al. 1994, Kinney et al. 1997). Many factors influence the morphological result, not least the timing of the insult, its impact upon crucial periods of brain growth and organisation, and the

TABLE 2.1
A timetable for hypoxic–ischaemic lesions in early life

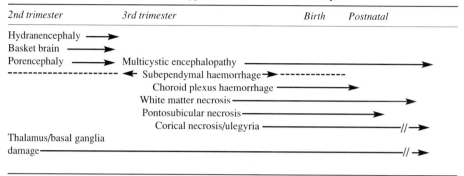

2nd trimester	3rd trimester	Birth	Postnatal

Hydranencephaly ⟶
Basket brain ⟶
Porencephaly ⟶ Multicystic encephalopathy ⟶
----------------------- ◂ Subependymal haemorrhage ➤ -------------
　　　　　　　　　　Choroid plexus haemorrhage ⟶
　　　　　　　　　　White matter necrosis ⟶
　　　　　　　　　　Pontosubicular necrosis ⟶
　　　　　　　　　　Corical necrosis/ulegyria ⟶ //➤
Thalamus/basal ganglia
damage ⟶ //➤

Dotted line indicates rarer occurence.

changing patterns of tissue response which parallel the maturation of the supporting glial cells. As a rule midgestational insults end in smooth-walled defects such as hydranencephaly or porencephaly, perhaps fringed by disorganised cortex, for the destruction may interfere with the later stages of neuroblast migration and by this time macrophages are already avid scavengers of necrotic tissue while astrocytic activity is absent. By the third trimester mature astrocytic responses are in place so multicystic ragged cavities are produced. This form of multicystic encephalopathy may also occur rarely in early postnatal life. Although global perfusion failure including that associated with intrauterine infections or as a complication of twinning might be expected to produce bilateral pathology, this is simply not the case. Explanations are usually not forthcoming, and markedly asymmetrical or strictly unilateral hemispheric involvement form the pathological basis of many cases of congenital hemiplegia. Often these infarcts are based on the territory of the middle cerebral artery, but only very rarely can direct evidence for arterial obstruction be adduced. Separately or combined with these headline-grabbing lesions there are also the various stigmata of birth injury, white and grey matter damage, haemorrhages and infarctions associated with birth asphyxia. In the context of surgical intervention for chronic unilateral epilepsy and hemiplegia the pathologist encounters the end stages of these processes (Figs 2.5, 2.6): cystic cavities in the white matter, shrunken gliotic convolutions of mushroom shape called ulegyria, mineralised neuronal debris, aberrant myelination following glial scars in cortex or basal grey matter (marbling).

CHRONIC POSTCONVULSIVE HEMIPLEGIA

Also known as hemiconvulsion-hemiplegia-epilepsy syndrome, the pathological changes in this rare complication of inadequately treated febrile convulsions or prolonged status epilepticus are much like those following perinatal hypoxic–ischaemic insult, a combination of atrophic cystic cortex and cavitated subcortical white matter (Fig 2.7).

22

Fig. 2.5. Extensive unilateral perinatal hypoxic–ischaemic destruction of the left hemisphere. Much of the centrum semi-ovale is destroyed, the digitate white matter is cystic while selective loss of deeper cortex has resulted in a mushroom-appearance of the convolutions, known as ulegyria.

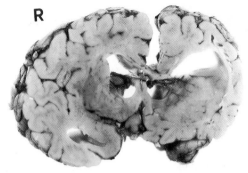

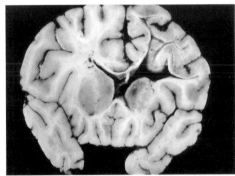

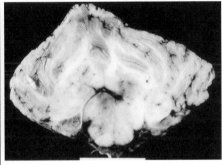

Fig 2.6. *(a)* A further example of unilateral perinatal hypoxic–ischaemic damage, principally to the white matter but also to the striatum *(b)* A horizontal section through the hindbrain reveals tiny ipsilateral pyramidal tract but hypertrophy of the contralateral tract.

Vascular lesions

Vasculopathy is rare in childhood. Exceptional instances of congenital berry aneurysm, or fusiform aneurysm associated with hypertension, present to the pathologist as massive fatal haemorrhage rather than infarctions of more restricted extent which are treatable and fortunately less rare in clinical practice. Arterio-venous malformations and cavernous haemangiomata are also rare in childhood. However, with the expansion of paediatric epilepsy surgery, examples of Sturge–Weber syndrome (Fig. 2.8) are increasingly encountered. Of course the stigmata of this phakomatosis are not always strictly unilateral, but in the vast majority of patients there is unilateral facial cutaneous vascular naevus and unilateral neurological deficit referable to unilateral meningeal venous angiomatosis associated with cortical atrophy and calcification.

Rasmussen syndrome

Despite marked histological resemblances to a low-grade chronic viral encephalitis, no causative agent has yet been convincingly demonstrated for this refractory unilateral seizure disorder despite modern investigation with molecular and immunohistochemical probes

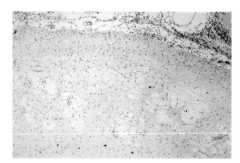

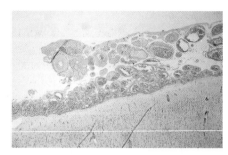

Fig. 2.7. Hemiplegia hemiconvulsion epilepsy syndrome. Complete destruction of the cortical ribbon.

Fig. 2.8. Sturge–Weber syndrome. The abnormal venous plexus in the leptomeninges is readily demonstrated with a reticulin silver impregnation.

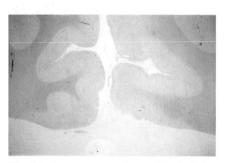

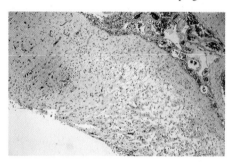

Fig. 2.9. Rasmussen syndrome: The inferior frontal cortex of left and right hemispheres from a fatal case. Note the remarkable sparing of the left hemispheric cortex while on the right side the cortical ribbon is thinned and shows mid-cortical cystic breakdown.

Fig. 2.10. A biopsy specimen in Rasmussen syndrome. Inflammatory changes may be patchy. On the left side of the figure intact cortical structure and nerve cells are evident but there is a neuronophagic nodule. By contrast the adjacent cortex to the right is completely disorganised, spongy gliotic and devoid of neurones.

(Honavar et al. 1992, 1997). Other suggested mechanisms include vascular immune complex deposition or circulating antibodies to glutamate receptor (GluR3) fusion protein (Rogers et al. 1994). Focal and partial complex seizures begin abruptly in childhood followed by progressive motor, visual and mental deficit. Although self limiting in some cases, the progressive cortical destruction may spread from an initial focus to involve the whole of one hemisphere (Fig. 2.9). Macroscopic changes vary from minimal to overt cortical atrophy. Microscopic changes include leptomeningeal chronic inflammatory infiltrate, and perivascular inflammatory cuffing, microglial nodules and neuronophagia in the cortex. The white matter may be affected to a lesser extent, and sometimes the basal ganglia also, but the brain stem, cerebellum or notably the contralateral cerebral hemisphere. Early on in the first year or two of the clinical disorder, inflammatory changes in surgical specimens can be quite subtle, but in more chronic cases cortical neurones and parenchyma are destroyed and replaced by a thin spongy gliotic remnant (Fig. 2.10).

Postscript

Epilepsy is a major clinical problem in children with hemiplegia, thus the morphological appearances of the hippocampus are of considerable pathogenetic interest. Published data are confusing in this area, but personal experience has provided ample evidence of the cooccurrence of major hippocampal involvement with temporal or extratemporal epileptogenic lesions (>15% of a large personal series of surgical resections undertaken for the relief of seizures). In particular, classical mesial temporal sclerosis may be present in patients with a great variety of other pathology including migration defects, infarcts, Sturge–Weber syndrome or Rasmussen syndrome.

REFERENCES

Duong T, De Rosa MJ, Poukens V, Vinters HV, Fisher RS. (1994) Neuronal cytoskeletal abnormalities in human cerebral cortical dysplasia. *Acta Neuropathologica,* **87,** 493–503.

Ellison D, Love S, Chimelli L, Harding, B., Lowe, J., Roberts, G., Vinters, H. (1998) *Neuropathology. A Reference Text of CNS Pathology.* London: Mosby.

Harding B, Copp AJ. (1997) Malformations. *In:* Graham DI, Lantos PL, editors.*Greenfield's Neuropathology. 6th edn.* London: Arnold, p. 387–533.

Harding BN. (1994) The Brain. *In:* Reed GB, Claireaux AE, Cockburn F, editors.*Diseases of the Fetus and Newborn. 2nd edn.* London: Chapman and Hall. p. 413–464.

Honavar M, Janota I, Polkey CE. (1992) Rasmussen's encephalitis in surgery for epilepsy. *Developmental Medicine and Child Neurology,* **34,** 3–14.

— Meldrum BS. (1997) Epilepsy. *In:* Graham DI, Lantos PL, editors.*Greenfield's Neuropathology. 6th edn.* London: Arnold. p 931–971.

Kinney HC, Armstrong DD, (1997) Perinatal Neuropathology. *In:* Graham DI, Lantos PL, editors.*Greenfield's Neuropathology. 6th edn.* London: Arnold. p. 537–600.

Rogers SW, Andrews PI, Gahring LC, Whisenand T, Cauley K, Crain B, Hughes TE, Heinemann SF, McNamara JO. (1994) Autoantibodies to glutamate receptor GluR3 in Rasmussen's encephalitis. *Science,* **265,** 648–651.

Rorke LB. (1992) Perinatal Brain Damage. *In:* Adams JH, Duchen LW, editors.*Greenfield's Neuropathology. 5th edn.* London: Arnold. p. 639–708.

Taylor DC, Falconer MA, Bruton CJ, Corsellis JAN. (1971) Focal dysplasia of the cerebral cortex in epilepsy. *Journal of Neurology, Neurosurgery and Psychiatry,* **34,** 369–387.

3
NEURORADIOLOGY

Lars-Martin Wiklund

To find the relation between pre-, peri- and postnatal events as the cause of cerebral palsy (CP) has been the objective of many clinical, neuropathological and neuroradiological studies. Clinical studies have been limited by the reliability of the clinical information. Neuropathological studies have been restricted by the limited number of cases considered, with often just the most severely affected being examined. Modern non-invasive neuroimaging techniques, such as computerized tomography (CT) and magnetic resonance imaging (MRI) have made it possible to perform neuroimaging in most patients. These modern techniques have contributed to the understanding of many CP syndromes such as hemiplegic CP – congenital hemiplegia – (Koch et al. 1980; Kulakowski and Larroche 1980; Michaelis et al. 1980; Cohen et al. 1981; Kotlarek et al. 1981; Pedersen et al. 1982; Claeys et al. 1983; Taudorf et al. 1984; Yokochi et al. 1985; Molteni et al. 1987; Wiklund et al. 1990, 1991a, b; Scher et al. 1991; Wiklund and Uvebrant 1991; Truwit et al. 1992; van Bogaert et al. 1992; Steinlin et al. 1993; Bouza et al. 1994a, b; Krägeloh-Mann et al. 1994, 1995; Niemann et al. 1994). This chapter will deal with CT and MRI in congenital hemiplegia.

The diagnosis of CP syndromes such as congenital hemiplegia is often made some months or even years after birth. Thus neuroradiology rarely documents the insult causing the impairment, but documents the resulting lesion. However, by correlating the morphological findings documented by neuroimaging with neuropathological knowledge it is often possible to characterize the lesions and to assess the time of insult as an adjunct in the etiological analysis (Michaelis et al. 1980; Barkovich and Truwit 1990; Scher et al. 1991; Wiklund et al. 1991a, b; Steinlin et al. 1993; Bouza et al. 1994a; Krägeloh-Mann et al. 1994; Niemann et al. 1994).

Why neuroimaging?
Although neuroimaging may not provide a clear pathway to specific treatment it has been found to be of increasing value. It provides evidence of the pathological basis for the impairments which may help in advising parents about causation and eventually about prognosis. It is a crucial part of the process by which epidemiological data can be developed into preventative strategies. It is also increasingly used in the medico-legal aspects of the subject (Volpe 1992).

Imaging in children with CP is imaging of manifest lesions which are at a chronic stage since CP, by definition, is a collection of chronic impairments. Hemiplegic impairments may be caused by any destructive lesion in the cortico-spinal system, anywhere between the cerebral cortex and the medulla. The spectrum of lesions shown by neuroradiology shows that congenital hemiplegia originates any time from early fetal life until the perinatal period.

CT is a sufficiently adequate method for documenting macroscopic lesions such as parenchymal defects. However, the range of projection and resolution options is limited and small lesions and subtle changes may elude detection. In many cases a CT of high quality may be able to differentiate between gray and white matter, but a more detailed assessment of the parenchyma of the brain is not possible. MRI is a more sensitive method of imaging and can look at more specific areas, with the potential to scan in any arbitrary projection and to reveal more subtle lesions in the brain parenchyma, e.g. gliosis, variations in myelination and subtle migration disorders.

The developing brain
During the first period of gestation, up to approximately 24 weeks', the development of the brain is determined by histogenesis and organogenesis. We can recognize the structure of a brain when the neuronal migration is essentially completed. However, there are important differences between the fetal and the mature brain. Pape and Wigglesworth (1979) stated, concerning the developing brain, that, "In many ways there are greater differences between the brain of a 28-week gestation infant and that of a 36 week infant, than there are between the brain of a three-month old baby and an adult." (p.vi) These differences include the vascular pattern, the metabolic demand in various regions and the density of various neurotransmittors which varies with the developmental stage. Circulation in the preterm period is predominantly periventricular in contrast to the circulation of the mature brain. The arterial watershed areas, thus vulnerable to ischemia, are located periventricularly, in contrast to the mature brain where those areas are located cortically/subcortically.

Thus lesional patterns after an insult to the developing brain are determined by the developmental stage of the brain.

Brain lesions in congenital hemiplegia
Although the spectrum of lesions in congenital hemiplegia is very wide, the morphological patterns seen as the end-stage after insults to the developing brain, could be divided into three main groups: cerebral malformations, periventricular lesions and cortical/subcortical lesions (Wiklund et al. 1990, Steinlin et al. 1993, Krägeloh-Mann et al. 1995, Sugimoto et al. 1995). These different patterns are important to recognize since they are good pointers to the timing of the insults to the brain. Cerebral malformations are indicators of a lesion of early fetal origin, up to a gestational age of approximately 24 weeks. Later insults – up to 34 weeks of gestational age – result in periventricular lesions. After a gestational age of 34 weeks the insult will cause a cortical/subcortical lesion.

CEREBRAL MALFORMATIONS
All malformations originate in early fetal life. The neuroblasts, which will create the cortex, originate in the germinal matrix, in the lateral wall of the ventricle. The neuroblasts start their migration to the surface of the brain during the 7th week of gestation. The migration is most intensive during the 3rd to the 5th month and is essentially ended during the 20th

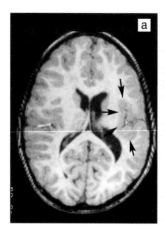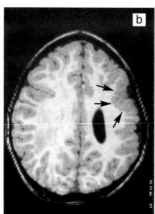

Fig. 3.1. *(a and b)* Boy aged 3 years with a right-sided hemiplegia. The boy was born at term and had no history of any pre- or perinatal event. MRI with an inversion recovery sequence shows in the left hemisphere a dysmorphic central sulcus surrounded by irregular and thickened cortex (see arrows) consistent with polymicrogyria.

to the 24th week. However, the germinal matrix, being the source of the glioblasts, is present until term.

Any insult during the period of neuronal migration may cause a migration disorder. These include agyria or lissencephaly in the early phase, schizencephaly and pachygyria later, and heterotopias and polymicrogyria in the late stage. The latter disorder can be caused up to the 30th week (Evrard et al. 1992). The associated clinical manifestations are dependent on the location and extension of the malformation. Unilateral and focal malformations may clinically be rather silent depending on the plasticity of the developing brain.

An early fetal origin of hemiplegia manifesting as a cerebral malformation was described in the 19th century (Heschl 1861). The most common malformations belong to the group of neuronal migration disorders (Wiklund et al. 1990) such as schizencephaly, focal pachygyria, heterotopia and polymicrogyria (Fig. 3.1) (Miller et al. 1984, Barkovich and Norman 1988, Wiklund et al. 1990, Truwit et al. 1992, Sebire et al. 1993). Also disorders of defective histogenesis, such as Sturge–Weber syndrome could be the cause of congenital hemiplegia (Wiklund et al. 1990). In the diagnosis of neuronal migration disorders it is extremely important to be able to differentiate between gray and white matter. The majority of these malformations are adequately documented by CT of good technical quality (Zimmerman et al. 1983, Buckley et al. 1989), although MRI is preferable (Barkovich et al. 1988).

PERIVENTRICULAR LESIONS
During the period of prematurity, i.e. from week 24 up to 34 of gestation, the most vulnerable part of the brain is the periventricular white matter, where the metabolic demand is highest because it is a vascular border zone at that time (Pape and Wigglesworth 1979). Thus insults during this period result predominantly in periventricular white matter lesions (Banker and Larroche 1962, DeReuck et al. 1972, Armstrong and Norman 1974, Shuman and Selednik 1980). Some factors which play a role in periventricular vulnerability are the presence of the germinal matrix; an immature vascular system; pressure-passive circulation which is

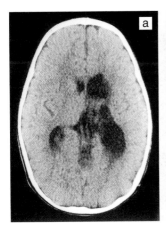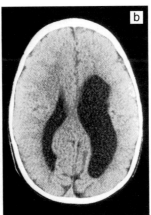

Fig. 3.2. *(a and b)* Boy aged 14 months with a right-sided hemiplegia. The boy was born preterm and had neonatally a periventricular hemorrhagic infarction documented with ultrasonography. CT shows a large left ventricle with a rather extensive defect in the entire periventricular white matter.

easily induced in the preterm; periventricular arterial border- and endzones; specific metabolic properties of the periventricular white matter during this period; and the actively differentiating and/or myelinating periventricular glial cells that are exceptionally vulnerable.

The cerebral cortex has a low metabolic rate during this period of development and is protected from circulatory disturbances by leptomeningeal anastomoses (Pape and Wigglesworth 1979, Volpe 1995). Thus the cortex is only affected by the most extensive lesions.

Periventricular lesions in congenital hemiplegia could represent end-stages of periventricular hemorrhagic infarctions (PHI) and periventricular leukomalacia (PVL).

PHI are predominantly seen in the very preterm infant (Volpe 1995). These lesions are often unilateral and seen as a ventriculomegaly, with significant loss of periventricular white matter (Fig. 3.2). Signs of gliotic scarring, manifested as a high T_2-signal in the periventricular white matter, are often lacking. This could be explained by the incapacity due to immaturity of the white matter to react with gliosis at the time of insult. T_2-weighted images could reveal deposition of periventricular hemosiderin (Takanashi et al. 1995).

The infants with PVL are mostly slightly more mature than those with PHI (Shuman and Selednik 1980). PVL is mostly bilateral with the clinical correlate of spastic diplegia, although it may also be seen in congenital hemiplegia (Wiklund et al. 1990). As in PHI there is a periventricular white matter reduction with irregular outline of the lateral ventricular wall. A peritrigonal location is common, thus having a close connection to the visual tract (Flodmark et al. 1990, Schenk-Rootlieb et al. 1994). In spite of a definite white matter reduction there is not always ventriculomegaly. A careful assessment of the thickness of the white matter is thus essential. Deep sulci with the depth of the sulci reaching almost to the ventricular wall may be diagnostic and can be seen quite well on CT (Flodmark et al. 1988) (Fig. 3.3). The diagnosis is more obvious with MRI since there is often a periventricular high T_2-signal including the immediate periventricular region as an indication of delayed myelination or gliotic scarring (Flodmark et al. 1989) (Fig. 3.4). Sometimes it is not possible to macroscopically differentiate between the end-stages of PHI and PVL (Volpe 1995). However, this differentiation is not so important from an etiological point of view. What is important is to make the diagnosis of a periventricular lesion, which occurs in the period of prematurity.

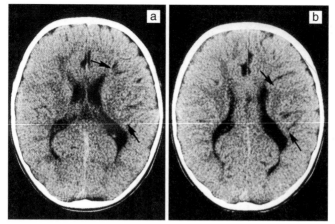

Fig. 3.3. *(a and b)* Girl aged 2 years, who was born at 30 weeks' gestational age and with an eventful perinatal history. The girl has a right-sided hemiplegia. CT shows reduction of the periventricular white matter in the left hemisphere. Note the deep sulci *(arrows)* and the close proximity of the cortical infoldings to the periventricular wall. The pathological correlate is unilateral periventricular leukomalacia.

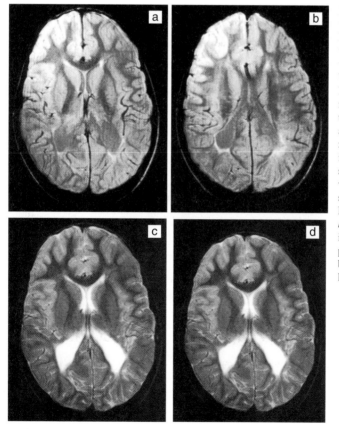

Fig. 3.4. Boy aged 7 years with a right-sided hemiplegia. MRI with *(a and b)* PD-weighted and *(c and d)* T$_2$-weighted images shows bilateral lesions. There is a loss of perventricular white matter dorsal and cranial of the occipital horns. There is an immediate periventricular zone with increased signal interpreted as gliotic scarring. That scarring is not visible on CT. The increased signal is best assessed on the PD-weighted images *(a and b)* where the signal from CSF is suppressed. The pathological correlate is bilateral periventricular leukomalacia.

30

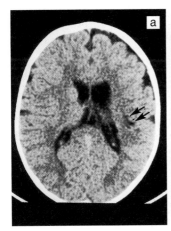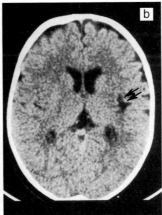

Fig. 3.5. *(a and b)* Boy aged 16 months with impairment of the function of his right hand and slightly of his leg. The boy was born at term and had no history of any pre- or perinatal event. CT shows a left-sided temporal subcortical hypodensity *(arrows)* and a discrete secondary widening of the subarachnoidal space. The finding is consistent with subcortical leukomalacia.

The periventricular watershed areas migrate peripherally to the subortical/cortical area when the arterial supply is maturing. Thus, between 34 and 38 weeks of gestation – the late preterm period – the subcortical areas are the most vulnerable to ischemia. The pathological correlate during that period is subcortical leukomalacia (SCL) (Takashima et al. 1978) (Fig. 3.5).

CORTICAL LESIONS
When the origin of the congenital hemiplegia is found to originate at term the resulting lesions predominantly have the appearance of ischemic infarctions of the adult brain, i.e. cortical infarctions (Wiklund et al. 1991b) (Fig. 3.6).

MISCELLANEOUS AND ASSOCIATED LESIONS
With MRI it has been possible to show diencephalic lesions in a large proportion of patients (Steinlin et al. 1993). These lesions are found as signal alterations in the diencephalon, including thalamus, basal ganglia, and caudate nucleus as well as the internal capsule, and could be primary or secondary lesions. Wallerian degeneration of the corticospinal tracts of the ipsilateral side may be seen as secondary to the periventricular as well as the cortical lesions (Bouza et al. 1994a). This degeneration may be manifested as a reduction in the volume of the basal ganglia, signal abberations in the internal capsule or as asymmetry of the upper brain stem. Cortical infarctions are often seen in combination with loss of volume of the surrounding parenchyma with the result of hemiatrophy (Wiklund et al. 1990).

Summary of brain lesions in congenital hemiplegia
The predominant lesions found in children with congenital hemiplegia correlated to time of insult are summarized in Table 3.1. We know that the hemiplegia is of a definite prenatal origin in a child with a cerebral malformation. The finding of a periventricular lesion is strong evidence of a prenatal injury in those born at term without obvious evidence of perinatal hypoxic–ischemic events (Wiklund et al. 1991b).

31

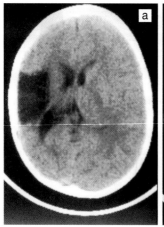 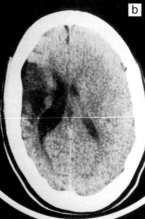

Fig. 3. 6. *(a and b)* Girl aged 8 years with a left-sided hemiplegia. Birth was at term (GA 41 wk). The pre- and perinatal history was uneventful except for prolonged labour. CT shows a cortical temporal infarction within the supply area of the right medial cerebral artery. Hemiatrophy of the right hemisphere is also noted.

In a population based Swedish CT study of 111 children with congenital hemiplegia (Table 3.2) it was shown that malformations were more frequent than previously thought (Wiklund et al. 1990). Every sixth patient had a cerebral malformation as the basis of their congenital hemiplegia, which is a similar proportion to a Swiss hospital-based MRI study (Steinlin et al. 1993). Periventricular lesions considered to represent periventricular hemorrhagic infarctions and periventricular leukomalacia was the most predominant finding. This result has later been reproduced in a MRI study (Niemann et al. 1994). Cortical infarctions were previously thought of as the most frequent finding in congenital hemiplegia, but turned out to be quite infrequent. Similar findings have later been confirmed by MRI studies (Steinlin et al. 1993). The proportion of cases with normal imaging in the Swedish material was relatively high but would be less if the study had been performed with MRI because of the greater sensitivity of this method (van Bogaert et al. 1992)

Although clinical hemiplegia tends to be associated with a unilateral lesion, bilateral lesions are seen in 12 to 24% of patients with hemiplegia (Wiklund et al. 1990, Steinlin et al. 1993). The contralateral lesions are frequently of the same type as the lesions causing the motor impairment. However, there are cases of hemiplegia caused by a malformation with a periventricular lesion in the contralateral hemisphere and vice versa (see Fig. 3.4).

Correlation of brain lesions and clinical manifestations
The morphological findings in congenital hemiplegia can be correlated to clinical manifestations (Wiklund and Uvebrant 1991).

MALDEVELOPMENTS
In the study by Wiklund and Uvebrant (1991) children with hemiplegia who had a cerebral maldevelopment had a hemiplegia that was predominantly arm dominated and they had growth impairment of the leg. Somewhat surprisingly a significant occurrence of epilepsy was not found in this study.

TABLE 3.1
Predominant brain lesions in congenital hemiplegia related to time of insult

Stage of development	Type of lesion
Early fetal life	Cerebral malformations
Very preterm	Periventricular hemorrhagic infarction (PHI)
Preterm	Periventricular leukomalacia (PVL)
Late preterm	Subcortical leukomalacia (SCL)
Term	Cortical infarctions

TABLE 3.2
Brain lesions in 111 patients with congenital hemiplegia.
CT findings (Wiklund et al. 1990)

CT findings	Preterm (n=28)	Term (n=83)
Maldevelopment	5	14
Periventricular lesion	14	33
Cortical/subcortical lesion	2	11
Miscellaneous	0	3
Normal	7	22

PERIVENTRICULAR LESIONS

Periventricular lesions correlated only with growth impairment of the leg. Lesions close to the frontal horn correlated with arm-dominated hemiplegia (Wiklund and Uvebrant 1991).

CORTICAL–SUBCORTICAL LESIONS

The children is this group were more likely to have a more severe total disability than other children with hemiplegia. They had significantly more impaired hand function, stereognosis, two-point discrimination and general motor function and they were also affected by facial weakness and epilepsy (Wiklund and Uvebrant 1991).

NORMAL FINDINGS

A normal CT was associated with significantly fewer impairments than in those children with hemiplegia who had a definite lesion.

There is often a poor correlation between the extent of the lesion and the severity of the impairment (Wiklund and Uvebrant 1991, Bouza et al. 1994b).

Choice of method of neuroimaging

Most brain lesions in congenital hemiplegia can be seen with CT. This method could easily be used for the screening of children with congenital hemiplegia since the availability of CT is good, it is a cheap method and the need for sedation is much less than for MRI. However, the examination should be completed with MRI in those cases when CT is normal or equivocal. MRI could be used as the primary method in children who may be examined without any sedation and when the access to MRI is very good. It is important to realize that neuroradiology can not visualize all lesions causing congenital hemiplegia. Even in children with severe impairments the result of neuroimaging may be normal. It now seems to be established practice that MRI has become the imaging modality of choice.

<small>TECHNICAL ASPECTS</small>
The whole brain should be scanned, from the foramen magnum up to the top of the convexity. To minimize the effect of partial volume the slices should not be thicker than 5 mm. There is rarely any need for contrast enhancement, either in CT or MRI.

CT
With CT the slices should be contiguous through the ventricles. It is hardly of any value to perform multiple projections with CT. In pediatric CT scanning it is always important to avoid unnecessary radiation. Thus, the gantry should be tilted more than in adult scanning so the eyes are not included in the scan. Since calcification of the calvarium in children is less than in adults it is important to use a specific pediatric algorithm. If the adult brain algorithm is used in a small child the attenuation of the cortex will be too high and the assessment of the cortex obstructed.

MRI
MRI should always include T_2-weighted sequences in at least two projections (axial and coronal). FLAIR is an excellent sequence to use to assess the periventricular white matter, since there is no signal from the spinal fluid. To obtain optimal anatomical resolution, including separation of gray and white matter, a heavily T_1-weighted sequence should be included (e.g. inversion recovery – IR). An interslice gap of 1 to 3 mm on MRI could be compensated by multiple projections, i.e. sagittal and coronal, in addition to the conventional axial.

Summary
It is the author's opinion that every child with congenital hemiplegia should be examined by brain scan using CT or MRI. The information obtained from neuroimaging provides an objective and reliable complement to clinical data. Patients, parents and physicians all benefit from this complementary information.

REFERENCES

Armstrong, D., Norman, M.G. (1974) Periventricular leukomalacia in neonates. Complications and sequelae. *Archives of Diseases of Childhood*, **49**, 367–375.
Banker, B.Q., Larroche, J-C. (1962) Periventricular leukomalacia of infancy. *Archives of Neurology*, **7**, 386–410.
Barkovich, A.J, Chuang, S.H., Norman, D. (1988) MR of Neuronal migrations anomalies. *American Journal of Radiology*, **9**, 179–187.
— Norman, D. (1988) MR Imaging of Schizencephaly. *American Journal of Neuroradiology*, **9**, 297–302.
— Truwit, C.L. (1990) Brain damage from perinatal asphyxia: Correlation of MR findings with gestational age. *American Journal of Neuroradiology*, **11**, 1087–1096.
Bouza, H., Dubowitz, L.M., Rutherford, M., Cowan, F., Pennock, J.M. (1994a) Late magnetic resonance imaging and clinical findings in neonates with unilateral lesions on cranial ultrasound. *Developmental Medicine and Child Neurology*, **36**, 951–964.

— Dubowitz, L.M.S., Rutherford, M., Pennock, J.M. (1994b) Prediction of outcome in children with congenital hemiplegia: A magnetic resonance imaging study. *Neuropediatrics, 25,* 60–66.

Buckley, A.R., Flodmark, O., Roland, E.H., Hill, A. (1989) Neuronal migration abnormalities can still be diagnosed by computed tomography. *Pediatric Neuroscience, 14,* 222–229.

Claeys, V., Deonna, T., Chrzanowski, R. (1983) Congenital hemiparesis: The spectrum of lesions. *Helvetia Pediatrica Acta, 38,* 493–455.

Cohen, M.E., Duffner, P.K. (1981) Prognostic indicators in hemiparetic cerebral palsy. *Annals of Neurolology, 9,* 353–357.

DeReuck, J., Chattha. A.S., Richardson, E.P. (1972) Pathogenesis and evolution of periventricular leukomalacia in infancy. *Archives of Neurology, 27,* 229–236.

Evrard, Ph., Miladi, N., Bonnier, C., Gressens, P. (1992) Normal and abnormal development of the brain. In: Rapin, I., Segalowitz, S.J., (Eds). *Handbook of Neuropsychology, Vol 6: Child Neuropsychology.* Amsterdam: Elsevier, p.11–44.

Flodmark, O., Roland, E.H., Hill, A., Whitfield, M.F. (1988) Periventricular leukomalacia: Radiologic diagnosis. *Radiology, 162,* 119–124.

— Jan, J.E., Wong, P.K.H. (1990) Computed tomography of the brains of children with visual impairment. *Developmental Medicine and Child Neurology, 32,* 611–620.

— Lupton, B., Li, D., Stimac, G.K., Roland, E.H., Hill, A., Withfield, M.F., Norman, M.G. (1989) MR imaging of periventricular leukomalaci in childhood. *American Journal of Neuroradiology 10,* 111–118.

Heschl, R. (1861) Ein neuer fall von porencephalie. *Vierteljahresschr Prakt Heikld (Prag) 72,* 102–104.

Koch, B., Brailler, D., Eng, G., Binder, H. (1980) Computerized tomography in cerebral–palsied children. *Developmental Medicine and Child Neurology, 22,* 595–607.

Kotlarek, F., Rodewig, R., Brull, D. (1981) Computed tomographic findings in congenital hemiparesis in childhood and their relation to etiology and prognosis. *Neuropediatrics, 12,* 101–108.

Krägeloh–Mann, I., Petersen, D., Hagberg, B., Michaelis, R. (1994) Magnetic resonance imaging in the timing of pathological events – a study in spastic cerebral palsy children. *In:* Lou, H.C., Greisen,G., Falck Larsen, J. (Eds) *Brain Lesions in the Newborn.* Copenhagen: Muncksgaard, p. 178–188.

— Petersen, D., Hagberg, G., Vollmer, B., Hagberg, B., Michaelis, R. (1995) Bilateral spastic cerebral palsy – MRI Pathology and origin. Analysis from a representative series of 56 cases. *Developmental Medicine and Child Neurology, 27,* 379–397.

Kulakowski, S., Larroche, J.–C. (1980) Cranial computerized tomography in cerebral palsy. An attempt at anatomo–clinical and radiological correlations. *Neuropediatrics, 11,* 339–353.

Michaelis, R., Rooschus, B., Dopfer, R. (1980) Prenatal origin of congenital spastic hemiplegia. *Early Human Development, 4,* 243–245.

Miller, G.M., Stears, J.C., Guggenheim, M.A., Wilkening, G.N. (1984) Schizencephaly: A clinical and CT study. *Neurology, 34,* 991–1001.

Molteni, B., Oleari, G., Fredrizzi, E. (1987) Relation between CT patterns, clinical findings and etiological factors in children born at term, affected by congenital hemiparesis. *Neuropediatrics, 18,* 75–80.

Niemann, G., Wakat, J-P., Krägeloh–Mann, I., Grodd, W., Michaelis, R. (1994) Congenital hemiparesis and periventricular leukomalacia: Pathogenetic aspects on magnetic resonance imaging. *Developmental Medicine and Child Neurology, 36,* 943–950.

Pape, K.E., Wigglesworth, J.S. (1979) *Haemorrhage, Ischaemia and the Perinatal Brain. Clinics in Developmental Medicine Nos. 69/70.* London: Spastics International Medical Publications. p. vi.

Pedersen, H., Taudorf, K., Melchior, J.C. (1982) Computed tomography in spastic cerebral palsy. *Neuroradiology, 23,* 275–278.

Schenk– Rootlieb, A.J.F., van Nieuwenhuizen, O., van Waes, P.F.G.M., van der Graaf, Y. (1994) Cerebral visual impairment in cerebral palsy: Relation to structural abnormalities of the cerebrum. *Neuropediatrics, 25,* 68–72.

Scher, M.S., Belfar, H., Martin, J., Painter, M.J. (1991) Destructive brain lesion of presumed fetal onset: antepartum causes of cerebral palsy. *Pediatrics, 88,* 898–906.

Sebire, G., Goutières, F., Tardieu, M., Landrieu, P., Aicardi, J. (1993) Study of 43 children affected with radiologically diagnosed extended brain gyral anomlies: Macrogyri and/or no visible gyri. Distinct clinical and electroencephalographical features according to neuroradiological patterns. *Neuropediatrics, 24,* 176.

Shuman, R.M., Selednik, L.J. (1980) Periventricular leukomalacia: A one-year autopsy study. *Archives of Neurology, 37,* 231–235.

Steinlin, M., Good, M., Martin, E., Benziger, O., Largo, R.H., Boltshauser, E. (1993) Congenital hemiplegia:

Morphology of cerebral lesions and pathogenetic aspects from MRI. *Neuropediatrics,* **24,** 224–229.

Sugimoto, T., Woo, M., Nishida, N., Araki, A., Hara, T., Yasuhara, A., Kobayashi, Y., Yamanouchi, Y. (1995) When do brain abnormalities in cerebral palsy occur? An MRI study. *Developmental Medicine and Child Neurology,* **37,** 285–292.

Takanashi, J., Sugita, K., Fujii, K., Niimi, H. (1995) Periventricular hemosiderin deposition in patients with congenital hemiplegia. *Developmental Medicine and Child Neurology,* **37,** 1016–1019.

Takashima, S., Armstrong, D.L., Becker, L.E. (1978) Subcortical leukomalacia – Relationship to development of the cerebral sulcus and its vascular supply. *Archives of Neurology,* **35,** 470–472.

Taudorf, K., Melchior, J.C., Pedersen, H. (1984) CT Findings in spastic cerebral palsy. Clinical actiological and prognostic aspects. *Neuropediatrics,* **15,** 120–124.

Truwit, C.L., Barkovich, A.J., Koch, T.K., Ferriero, D.M. (1992) Cerebral palsy: MR findings in 40 patients. *American Journal of Neuroradiology,* **13,** 67–78.

van Bogaert, P., Baleriaux, D., Christope, C., Szliwowski, H.B. (1992) MRI of patients with cerebral palsy and normal CT scan. *Neuroradiology,* **34,** 52–56.

Volpe, J.J. (1992) Value of MR in definition of the neuropathology of cerebral palsy in vivo. *American Journal of Neuroradiology,* **13,** 79–83. (Commentary).

— (1995) *Neurology of the Newborn. 2nd edn,* Philadelphia: WB Saunders.

Wiklund, L-M., Uvebrant, P., Flodmark, O. (1990) Morphology of cerebral lesions in children with congenital hemiplegia: A study with computed tompography. *Neuroradiology,* **32,** 179–186.

— — (1991) CT morphology in correlation to clinical findings in hemiplegic cerebral palsy. *Developmental Medicine and Child Neurology,* **33,** 512–523.

— — Flodmark, O. (1991a) Computed tomography as an adjunct in etiological analysis of hemiplegic cerebral palsy, I: Children born preterm. *Neuropediatrics,* **22,** 50–56.

— — — (1991b) Computed tomography as an adjunct in etiological analysis of hemiplegic cerebral palsy, II: Children born at term. *Neuropediatrics,* **22,** 121–128.

Yokochi, K., Kitazumi, E., Enomoto, S., Yokochi, A., Kodama, K. (1985) The computed tomographic findings of hemiplegic cerebral palsy. *Brain and Development,* **7,** 168.

Zimmerman, R.A., Bilanuk, L.T., Grossman, R.I. (1983) Computed tomography in migratory disorders of human brain development. *Neuroradiology,* **25,** 257–263.

4
A NEW MRI-BASED CLASSIFICATION

Gerhard Niemann

Hemiparesis which has its origin pre- or perinatally represents a classic type of the group of disorders called cerebral palsy (CP). The underlying causes of the cerebral palsies have been under discussion for about 150 years.

It is not possible to determine the underlying causes of congenital hemipareses as long as they are considered as an homogeneous group, i.e. as one nosological entity. In fact, congenital spastic hemipareses only have in common the unilateral motor disability reflecting the involvement of the pyramidal tract system. The pathogenesis and aetiology of pyramidal tract damage seem to be completely heterogeneous.

It is necessary, therefore, to establish subgroups which should be analysed separately in nosological terms. A new classification based on magnetic resonance imaging (MRI) is particularly useful as it can indicate both the pathogenesis and timing of the lesion.

The system was used to test the hypotheses that: (1) congenital hemipareses form a very heterogeneous group in terms of the underlying cause; (2) different patterns of lesion reflect different pathogenetic events and different times when these events may have occurred; (3) MRI is the method of choice in defining underlying lesion patterns; (4) grouping according to criteria based on the results of imaging is of relevance to the clinical outcome.

Patients

The individuals chosen for the study were patients of the author's department who were born between January 1974 and December 1995. The patients had all been diagnosed with hemiparesis (for definition see below) which was confirmed after the first year of life (diagnosis between the 2nd and 16th year of age; for reexamination see details below). There was no evidence in any patient that the hemiparesis was caused after the perinatal period (that means the term 'congenital' is not used in its strictest sense of a problem linked to a genetic origin – a definition which is in accordance with the literature).

With the help of the database, 205 patients with congenital hemiparesis could be identified – 77 girls and 128 boys (37.6 and 62.4%). There were 57 (27.8%) preterm infants, 143 born at term (70%), and three were born after 42 weeks of gestation. There was no information concerning gestational age for two patients.

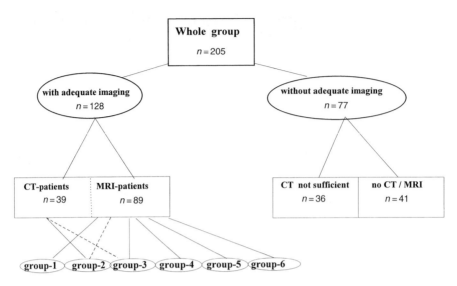

Fig. 4.1. The classification of patients: grouping according to MRI and CT.

Method

MEDICAL RECORDS AND DATABASE

Sex, gestational age, affected side, severity of hemiparesis, associated problems (cognitive development, epilepsy) as well as pre- and perinatal data were obtained from medical records and entered in a database.

Sixty-eight patients were reexamined clinically and by MRI. We tried to reexamine all patients at the age of 7 to 18 years in whom no MRI was done and in whom the CT did not reveal a lesion which was sufficient to explain the unilateral motor involvement (for grouping see below). It seems justified to include a subgroup who had 'only' a CT scan since we would not expect any additional information from MRI concerning the underlying cause if CT had already revealed a lesion which sufficiently explained the hemiparesis (i.e. a defect in the territory of the middle cerebral artery of some malformation patterns like in Sturge–Weber syndrome). This was confirmed by the experience of the author and his coworkers in some cases where CT and MRI were done. No additional information was gained by MRI in these cases. It is true that especially the group with lesions consistent with an infarction of the middle cerebral artery could be slightly overrepresented. Thus the relative proportions of our groups can not be seen as strictly representative.

GROUPING AND SCORING

The patients were divided into two groups, one with and one without adequate imaging. The following patients were judged as having had adequate imaging:(1) all patients who had had MRI ($n = 89$); (2) patients with a CT finding i.e. cortical–subcortical lesion in the territory of the middle cerebral artery explaining the motor disability ($n = 39$)(see group 2 finding below).

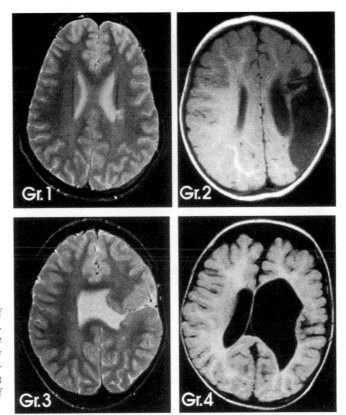

Fig. 4.2. MRI examples of the four main groups (1–4). (All photographs in the figures are reporoduced by kind permission of Professor Dr Voigt, Department of Radiology, University of Tübingen, Germany.

These 128 patients (62% of the whole group) could be further subdivided into groups 1 to 6 (Fig. 4.1). Only these patients were analysed in a more detailed manner.

The 77 patients without adequate imaging could be further subdivided into two groups: 41 patients without any imaging and 36 patients with CT findings which did not meet the above-mentioned criteria.

The classification of imaging results were (Fig. 4.2.):
• group 1: periventricular hyperintense lesions in T_2-weighted images
• group 2: cortical–subcortical lesion in the territory of the middle cerebral artery (CT or MRI)
• group 3: malformation patterns
• group 4: reduction of the periventricular white matter, enlargement of the ventricle (more than one-third of the hemisphere diameter) on MRI
• group 5: MRI finding did not meet criteria of groups 1, 2, 3, 4
• group 6: normal MRI

In order to assess the relation between pathology and function it was necessary to give a score to the motor disability. Therefore, we developed the following scoring system

TABLE 4.1
Motor disability score

	Stage 1 (mild)	Stage 2 (moderate)	Stage 3 (severe)	Stage 4 (very severe)
Upper extremity	Fine finger manipulation only mildly impaired	Fine finger manipulation significantly impaired	Fine finger manipulation impossible; hand function preserved	No grasping – (only 'helper') function
	(pincer grasp, turning a coin between the first three fingers)	(turning a coin impossible, but can lace one's shoes or pull on socks)	(holding or grasping a bottle or a door handle)	
Lower extremity	Primary ground contact by heel or plantigrade (rolling mechanism slightly impaired)	Primary ground contact by forefoot then plantigrade	Walking on forefoot; plantigrade position only when standing	Walking and standing on forefoot

describing the functional involvement of upper and lower limbs separately (Table 4.1). By this method, the hemiparesis could be judged to be arm or leg dominated.

The score was applied prospectively to the 44 patients who were reexamined and to the remaining patients when unequivocal data were obtained from the records.

MRI

MRI was performed on a whole-body tomograph working at 1.5 Tesla (Siemens Magnetom, Erlangen, Germany). The imaging protocol consisted of obtaining one set of sagittal and two sets of axial T_1-weighted images, as well one set of axial and coronal T_2-weighted images, all with spin-echo sequences (256×56 matrix, one acquisition, 4 mm slice thickness, 4 mm gap). For T_1-weighted images, the repetition time (RT) was 600 ms and the echo time (ET) was 15 ms. For T_2-balanced and T_2-weighted images, a double spin-echo sequence with motion suppression by gradient rephasing was used with a RT of 2000 ms and ET of 45 and 90 ms.

STATISTICS

Statistical analysis was performed for descriptive purposes, using StatXact-Turbo program (CYTEL Software Corporation, Cambridge, MA, USA). Continuous variables were described by use of statistical characteristics (means, standard deviations). Discrete variables were described as counts and percentages. To compare the distribution of discrete variables between two or more subgroups of patients, Fisher exact tests and χ^2 tests were used. To compare the distribution of continuous or ordinal scaled variables in two subgroups of patients or between two measures in one group the Wilcoxon test was used. Data are presented with nominal two-tailed exact p values (unadjusted for multiple comparisons).

Definitions

CONGENITAL HEMIPARESIS

We are dealing here with the congenital subgroup of so-called hemiplegic or hemiparetic CP only, which is defined as a unilateral motor disability. The decisive criterion for the diagnosis of 'hemiparesis' is functional disability, not individual neurological impairment (World Health Organization 1980). This definition contains the absence of any motor disability on the other side – but not of any neurological signs. There should be no evidence that the hemiparesis could have been caused after the perinatal period. The diagnosis was made by an experienced doctor in the author's department at the Kinderklinik, Tübingen, Germany.

GESTATIONAL AGE

Preterm means a gestational age < 38 weeks'; very preterm < 32 weeks' gestation.

LEARNING DISABILITY

Most of the patients did not have formal psychological assessment of cognitive function. Learning disability was assumed when the child did not attend mainstream school or age-appropriate mental development could be excluded by assessment by a paediatric neurologist in the author's department.

Results and discussion

GROUP 1

A group 1 lesion was defined as a hyperintense lesion in the periventricular white matter. This was the most common finding (36 patients = 28% of the group with adequate imaging). The ratio of 2.3:1 (term:preterm) is nearly the same as the ratio in the whole hemiparetic collective and the group with adequate imaging. But it is different from the ratio in groups 2 and 3 with the clearer predominance of term infants.

The symptomatology was arm dominated in seven children, leg dominated in 11 children; and in 16 patients upper and lower limbs were equally affected. Two patients could not be assessed. The periventricular site of the lesion did not correspond necessarily to a more severe disability of the lower than the upper limb – which is what could have been expected because of the somatotopic organization of the pyramidal tract system. Nevertheless, the ratio of leg-dominated paresis was higher than in the groups 2, 3 and 4 (32% versus 7, 5, and 18% in the other groups) ($p = 0.0266$ and 0.0137 and 0.3337). This appears to underline the closeness to the children with spastic diplegia.

The clinical scoring of 24 reexamined patients revealed that the majority ($n = 20$) had a moderate or mild disability of the upper and lower limbs. Compared to group 2, involvement of the hand (not of the foot) was significantly mild ($p = 0.0006$). Mental development could be assessed in 34 of the 36 patients. Only 15% had learning disability, which is a low rate in comparison with group 2 ($p = 0.0714$), group 3 ($p = 0.0001$) and group 4 ($p = 0.0489$). Only one patient had an epileptic disorder. According to the EEG findings it was a syndrome with continuous spike waves during slow sleep.

Exact analysis of the lesion patterns (within this group) was performed in 24 patients who could be clinically reexamined. MRI provided evidence of lesions especially in the

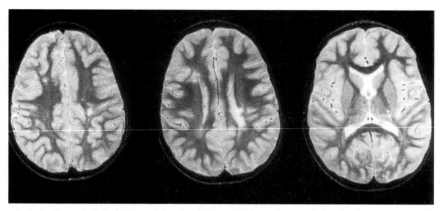

Fig. 4.3. Group 1 finding. T_2-weighted axial images; hyperintense lesion in the centrum semiovale, lateral to the ventricle and in the internal capsule (boy at the age of 15 y, born at term).

centrum semiovale and the periventricular region of the dorsal part of the lateral ventricle (cella media) (Fig. 4.3) (Niemann et al. 1994). The exact site and size of the lesion (within this group) did not correlate to the clinical outcome. Neuroimaging showed in 15 of the 25 term infants a unilateral lesion and in the other 10 a bilateral periventricular lesion. In contrast, in preterm infants there was a predominance of bilateral, and often more extensive signal abnormalities (Fig. 4.4). Four of the seven subjects born moderately preterm and three of the four very preterm infants had evidence of such a lesion.

The data from our department compared well with those of published MRI reports on (mostly preterm) children with spastic diplegia (Koeda et al. 1990, Konishi et al. 1990, Keeney et al. 1991, Lipper et al. 1991, Yokochi et al. 1991, van Bogaert et al. 1992, Krägeloh-Mann et al. 1992, Truwit et al. 1992, Flodmark et al. 1998). Therefore, we conclude that in both groups there is a similar pathogenesis – which could be ischaemia occurring between the 28th and 36th week of gestation (Krägeloh-Mann et al. 1994, 1995; Volpe 1995).

In contrast to the group with spastic diplegia the children in this study were mostly born at term. If there is a common pathogenesis (of spastic diplegia and hemiparesis with the group 1 pattern) we have to assume that the lesion is acquired prenatally in most of the hemiparetic patients. Perhaps the bilateral MRI lesions (though unilateral disability) being commoner in preterm infants, indicate linkage to preterm diplegia.

GROUP 2

Of the group with adequate imaging 32 patients (25%) had a cortical–subcortical lesion – a pattern which can be visualized by MRI and by CT and which, since the introduction of CT about 20 years ago, is well known as one of the main patterns of lesion (Koch et al. 1980, Michaelis et al. 1980, Kotlarek et al. 1981, Claeys et al. 1983, Molteni et al. 1987, Wiklund et al. 1990, Wiklund and Uvebrant 1991). Figure 4.5 shows a typical example. Usually, the pathogenesis behind this finding is regarded as an arterial thromboembolic ischemic event in the area of the middle cerebral artery (Clark and Linell 1954, Cocker et

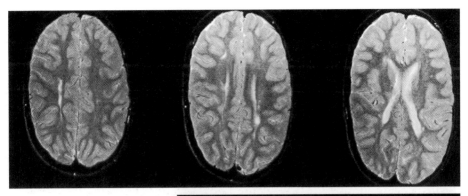

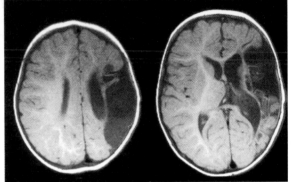

Fig. 4.4. *(above)* Group 1 finding. T_2-weighted axial images; bilateral lesions in the centrum semiovale and periventricular (boy at the age of 15 y, born at 35 wk gestation, sepsis, ventilation for 26 days).

Fig. 4.5. *(right)* Group 2 finding. T_1-weighted axial images; cortical—subcortical lesion in the territory of the middle cerebral artery (boy at the age of 8 mo, born at term).

al. 1965, Barmada et al. 1979, Mantovani and Gerber 1984, Asindi et al. 1988).

The distribution of gestational age (29 term children and three preterm) is different from group 1 (and from the distribution in the whole collective with adequate imaging) with significantly more term patients ($p = 0.0386$) – which is in accordance with other published data (Uvebrant 1988, Steinlin et al. 1993). It is suggested that this lesion type depends on a more mature pattern of vascularization, which takes place near term (DeReuck 1971, 1984; Barkovich and Truwit 1990; Allan and Riviello 1992; Volpe 1995).

As known from other reports (Wiklund et al. 1990, Steinlin et al. 1993, Khaw et al. 1994) we found more right-sided ($n = 23$) than left-sided ($n = 9$) pareses especially in this group (which could be due to anatomic differences between the left arteria carotis communis and the right truncus brachiocephalicus (Coker et al. 1988).

As mentioned above the disability of the upper limbs only was more severe than in group 1 ($p = 0.0006$) – which was reported by Molteni and colleagues too (Molteni et al. 1987). There was no difference regarding the involvement of the lower limbs between the groups. In 22 individuals we found an arm-dominated and in two subjects a leg-dominated paresis. In three patients there was no difference concerning the severity of motor disability between upper and lower limbs, and in five patients we were not able to assess the severity as the data material did not allow a definite grading.

Ten of the 27 patients who could be assessed had learning disability, which is a higher number than in group 1; seven of 27 patients had epileptic seizures – reflecting the handicap of this group (Uvebrant 1988, Süssová et al. 1990, Vargha-Khadem et al. 1992). Thus the comparison between the groups indicate that the imaging results indeed have prognostic value (Kotlarek et al. 1981, Claeys et al. 1983).

Generally, the lesion pattern in group 2 is regarded as the result of a focal ischaemic stroke in the area of the middle cerebral artery (Clark and Linell 1954, Cocker et al. 1965, Barmada et al. 1979, Mantovani and Gerber 1984, Asindi et al. 1988, Scher et al. 1991). In most cases the aetiology of this stroke in newborn infants is still obscure. We performed a study with eight affected patients from group 2 (age range 2 to 15 years). A detailed history including maternal and familial data was obtained. Duplex sonography was performed and biochemical parameters were analysed in all these patients and their mothers. There were no convincing hints of a prenatal (for instance, infectious, traumatic or toxic) origin. Also the history of the perinatal period could not explain the infarction. Neonatal epileptic seizures (in three patients) could perhaps indicate the time of the infarction, but do not explain the aetiology (Allan and Riviello 1992). Duplex sonography revealed no anatomic variants of intra- or extracerebral arteries (for method see Schöning et al. 1993). Haemostasiological results were within normal limits – except the (IgM-) antiphospholipid antibodies, which were present in six of the eight families (patient or mother). This could indicate a disposition for a thromboembolic event (Silver et al. 1992, Devilat et al. 1993, Angelini et al. 1994, Göbel 1994, Korte et al. 1994, Ravelli et al. 1994, Schöning et al. 1994, Dewitt 1995).

GROUP 3

Imaging in 27 patients (21% of the group with adequate imaging) showed evidence of an underlying malformation (nine patients with unilateral schizencephaly [Fig. 4.6], five patients with Sturge–Weber syndrome, six patients with hemiatrophy in part with cortical dysplasia [Fig. 4.7] and seven other malformation features).

Aetiopathogenetically these disorders are heterogeneous and, therefore, a synopsis of clinical parameters does not seem appropriate. (The cognitive development was frequently impaired, which was especially true for the patients with a disorder of proliferation or cortical organization including Sturge–Weber syndrome. Thirteen patients had epileptic disorder – nine of these with Sturge–Weber syndrome or cortical dysplasia. Patients with unilateral schizencephaly, however, showed a relatively benign outcome with regards to epilepsy (only two children had fits) and cognitive development (four children had learning disability). This is a suprisingly low rate of associated problems compared with the data published about patients with bilateral clefts (Barkovich and Kjos 1992).

The data of the author and his coworkers support the role of very early acquired lesions in the hemiparetic subgroup of CP (Wiklund et al. 1990, Steinlin et al. 1993). Therefore, analyses of the incidence of CP in relation to perinatal medicine have to take into account that a considerable proportion of the unilateral type of hemiplegia can not be influenced by perinatal care. Some of these malformation patterns are visible only by MRI (Barkovich and Klos 1992, Barth 1992, van Bogaert et al. 1992). Thus the importance of this technique is emphasized.

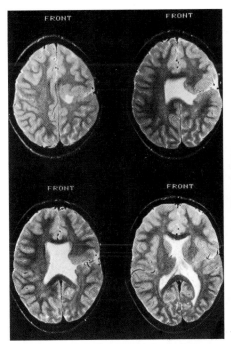

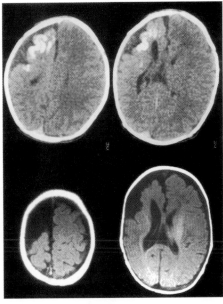

Fig. 4.7. Group 3 finding: CT with chalky signal (calcification) in the frontal region at the age of 5 d; T_1-weighted axial images provide the atrophy at the age of 4 mo; cortical dysplasia not identical to Sturge–Weber syndrome (girl, born at term).

Fig. 4.6. Group 3 finding: T_2-weighted axial images; unilateral schizencephaly (boy at the age of 12 y, born at term).

GROUP 4

This group is not yet characterized explicitly as having one of the main lesion patterns underlying congenital hemipareses. Up to now patients with these imaging features have been put together with the patients with periventricular lesions (Kotlarek et al. 1981, Wiklund et al. 1990). However, it seems that there is a difference concerning the underlying pathogenesis between the group 1 pattern in this study (often associated with mild ventricular enlargement) and group 4 with severe myelin defect (Fig. 4.8).

Eighteen patients (14.1% of the group with adequate imaging) had evidence of a group 4 pattern. There were six term and 12 preterm children. The gestational age is significantly lower in this group than in group 1 ($p = 0.0189$) or in group 2 ($p = 0.0001$). Seven of the 12 preterm children were born before 32 weeks of gestation. The motor disability of the upper limbs was graded on average as moderate, and of the lower limbs as mild or moderate. This indicates no major difference to group 1, but a less severely impaired motor function in comparison with group 2. In contrast to this relatively benign outcome with regards to motor function there was a high percentage (46%) of children with learning disability. Only two patients had epileptic seizures. This suggests that the influence of epileptogenesis on cognitive development is not considerable. Perhaps early damage of the germinal zone with its growing glial cells has consequences for thalamocortical connections and can explain the high

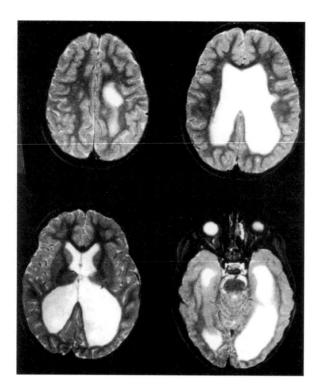

Fig.4.8. Group 4 finding. T_2-weighted axial images; myelin reduction and enlargement of the ventricle (boy at the age of 3y, born at 32 wk of gestation).

percentage of children with learning disability in this group (Volpe 1996a).

The following data and hypotheses support the author's view that this lesion pattern reflects a haemorrhagic event: (1) From eight patients in group 4 signs of neonatal bleeding are reported. We were able to visualize the postpartum haemorrhage by ultrasound sonography in three children. The MRI – performed later on – revealed a typical group 4 lesion pattern (Fig. 4.9).

(2) Preterm infants, especially very preterm children, are predisposed to haemorrhage (Beverley et al. 1984, Volpe 1989a, Rademaker et al. 1994). In our group 4, distribution of gestational age is clearly weighted towards these very preterm children.

(3) The severe and unilateral destruction of white matter is most compatible with a posthaemorrhagic lesion – which is not true for ischaemic events (Barkovich and Truwit 1990, Krägeloh-Mann et al. 1994).

(4) The vulnerability of the germinal zone especially in very preterm children could explain the ventricular enlargement and malformation. Most of the subependymal and intraventricular haemorrhages in these children occur in the first few hours or first 2 days of life and are followed by any involvement of parenchymal tissue (Beverley et al. 1984; Volpe 1995, 1996b). Volpe hypothesized that the intraventricular haemorrhage leads to venous infarction (Volpe 1989 a, b; 1995). Neuropathological data support this view (Takashima et al. 1986). Therefore, 'periventricular haemorrhagic infarction' is typically associated with

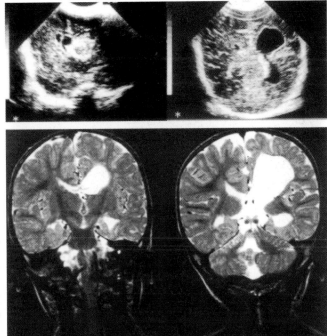

Fig 4.9. Group 4 finding. Ultrasound sonography at the age of 7 days and 4 months (the hemorrhage occurred after the second day of life); T$_2$-weighted coronal images at the age of 1½y (twin, born at 24 wk of gestational age.

intraventricular bleeding (Volpe 1989a, 1995, 1996b) and that is why the close relation of the periventricular white matter damage to the ventricle is not suprising. In most cases unilateral or asymmetric lesions develop (Guzzetta et al. 1986), and these are of course highly compatible with a unilateral motor problem.

Epidemiological analysis indicated 20 years ago that the prevalence of congenital hemipareses might be stable (Hagberg 1979). This was interpreted as a predominance of prenatal origins which could not be influenced by modern perinatal medicine (Michaelis et al. 1980, Michaelis and Niemann 1995). On the other hand, two papers recently reported an increase in the number of patients with hemipareses especially in the low gestational age group of children with CP. Stanley and Watson (1992) pointed out that in Western Australia hemipareses is the most common type of CP among very preterm children (< 1000 g birthweight). Pharoah and coworkers confirmed this tendency and reported an incidence of nearly 25 hemiparetic patients per 1000 live births among children with a birthweight of less than 1500 g (Pharoah et al. 1990). However, in both of these papers there is no description of the underlying lesion.

Our data suggest that there is not an increase in the numbers of congenital hemipareses as a whole but an increase in the numbers of patients with a group 4 type lesion. Very preterm children are showing increasing survival (Hagberg et al. 1989, Bushan et al. 1993) – but often with neurological (e.g. hemiparetic) and psychoorganic problems.

47

GROUP 5

Seven patients, four born at term and three preterm formed this group (5.6% of the group who had adequate imaging). One of these patients resembled the preterm children of group 1. He had evidence of a periventricular lesion extending to the subcortical white matter. Perhaps this represented an ischaemic event of a more mature vascularisation (37 weeks of gestation). Two other patients showed multiple or bilateral lesions with an extension to the subcortical region, a pattern of lesion also compatible with an ischaemic pathogenesis. Haemorrhages could be responsible for the lesions in the four remaining children in this group. Two patients had additional signs of a migration disorder (schizencephaly), but the hemiparesis could not be clearly attributed to this.

In this heterogeneous group, vascular damage seems to predominate as in group 1 and 2. The small amount of subjects in this group underlines the legitimacy of our classification.

GROUP 6

Eight children (one preterm) had normal MRI findings (6.3% of the patients with adequate imaging). Only two of these (1.6% of the patients with adequate imaging) had hemiparesis when reexamined at the age of 4 to 11 years. These data lead to the suggestion that the functional disability especially of the upper limbs will be mild when the MRI is normal (Niemann et al. 1996). Evidence of lesions on MRI seems to be correlated with the persistence of hemiparetic symptoms.

Six patients of this group, who still had signs of hemiparesis between the ages of 2 and 7 did not have any functional disability later on. The follow-up examinations in our department were carried out 7 to 14 years later. In this collective even those young people in whom a right hemiparesis had been diagnosed developed a contralateral handedness although there was no family history of left-handedness at all. This indicates that there was indeed a functional relevant unilateral cerebral disorder in the first few years of life. In addition, parents and patients did remember that their child had previously experienced a motor disability (Niemann et al. 1996).

Our study complements the results reported by Taudorf and colleagues, who carried out follow-up studies which consisted of clinical neurological examination and computed tomography on 17 patients who had previously been diagnosed with CP (Taudorf et al. 1986). The diagnosis of hemiparesis was made in one of their patients only, at the age of 6 months. Only 1 year later, no such disability was present. In our opinion, there is a grey area between 'remittent CP' and 'transitory neurological finding'. It is well known that neurological abnormalities in the first months of life often remit, not just in cases of preterm birth and perinatal asphyxia (Drillien 1972, Nelson and Ellenberg 1982, Piper et al. 1988, Michaelis et al. 1993). In view of this, we must avoid making a hasty diagnosis of CP, with its implication of lasting functional disabilities. The constellation of a mild and non-arm-dominated paresis and of a normal MRI indicates that a remission is possible in later childhood years. We conclude that some children 'outgrow' a hemiparetic disability, even in later childhood years. In our patient group this happened between the ages of 3 and 10. We further propose that MRI may be useful in distinguishing between transitory and persistent hemiparesis.

Summary

Due to of its sensitivity and specificity MRI is the method of first choice when investigating the cause of an unexplained congenital hemiparesis. Some lesion patterns can be detected only using this technique.

Different lesion patterns represent different pathogenetic events and the different times when these events may have occurred.

A nosological classification of congenital hemipareses should be based on these imaging criteria. The following differences between the established groups support this approach:

• gestational age: term infants predominate in group 2 and 3; very preterm infants in group 4;

• side of hemiparesis: left-hemisphere lesions predominate in group 2;

• motor disability: severe functional problems of the upper extremity are frequent in group 2; leg-dominated symptoms are frequent in group 1 only;

• associated problems: learning disability is very frequent in group 3, relatively frequent in group 2, and rare in group 1 patients;

• pre- and perinatal risk factors: perinatal problems are relevant especially in group 4.

With regards to aetiology, clinical outcome and epidemiology (Mutch et al. 1992) further investigation of these groups should be done separately. This approach could offer new insight into aetiopathogenesis and help to develop strategies for prophylaxis and intervention.

ACKNOWLEDGEMENT

Thanks are due to Professor Dr Voigt, Head of the Department of Neuroradiology; to Professor Dr Grodd and Dr Wakat for their cooperation and to C Meisner, Department of Medical Information Processing.

REFERENCES

Allan, W., Riviello, J. (1992) Perinatal cerebrovascular disease in the neonate. *Pediatric Clinics of North America* **39**, 621–650.

Angelini, L., Ravelli, A., Caporali, R., Rumi, V., Nardocci, N., Martini, A. (1994) High prevalence of antiphospholipid antibodies in children with idiopathic cerebral ischemia. *Pediatrics,* **94**, 500–503.

Asindi, A.A., Stephenson, J.B., Young, D.G. (1988) Spastic hemiparesis and presumed prenatal embolisation. *Archives of Diseases in Childhood,* **63**, 68–69.

Barkovich AJ, Truwit C. (1990) Brain damage from perinatal asphyxia: Correlation of MR findings with gestational age. *American Journal of Neuroradiology,* **11**, 1087–96.

— Kjos, B. (1992) Schizencephaly: Correlation of clinical findings with MR characteristics. *American Journal of Neuroradiology,* **13**, 85–94.

Barmada, M.A., Moossy, J., Shuman, R.M. (1979) Cerebral infarcts with arterial occlusion in neonates. *Annals of Neurology,* **6**, 495–502.

Barth, P.G. (1992) Schizencephaly and nonlissencephalic cortical dysplasias. *American Journal of Neuroradiology,* **13**, 104–106.

Beverley, D., Chance, G., Coates, C. (1984) Intraventricular haemorrhage - timing of occurrence and relationship to perinatal events. *British Journal of Obstetrics and Gynaecology,* **91**, 1007–1013.

Bushan, V., Paneth, N., Kiely, J. (1993) Impact of improved survival of very low birth weight infants on recent secular trends in the prevalence of cerebral palsy. *Pediatrics,* **91**, 1094–1100.

Claeys, V., Deonna, T., Chrzanowski, R. (1983) Congenital hemiparesis: the spectrum of lesions. A clinical and computerized tomographic study of 37 cases. *Helvetica Paediatrica Acta,* **38**, 439–455.

Clark, R.M., Linell, E.A. (1954) Case report: Prenatal occlusion of the internal carotid artery. *Journal of Neurology, Neurosurgery and Psychiatry,* **17**, 295–297.

Cocker, J., George, S.W., Yates, P.O. (1965) Perinatal occlusion of the middle cerebral artery. *Developmental Medicine and Child Neurology*, **7**, 235–243.

Coker, S., Beltran, R., Myers, T., Hmura, L. (1988) Neonatal stroke: description of patients and investigation into pathogenesis. *Pediatric Neurology*, **4**, 219–223.

DeReuck J. (1971) The human periventricular arterial blood supply and the anatomy of cerebral infarctions. *European Neurology*, **5**, 321–334.

— (1984) Cerebral angioarchitecture and perinatal brain lesions in premature and full-term infants. *Acta Neurologica Scandinavica* **70**, 391–395.

Devilat, M., Toso, M., Morales, M. (1993) Childhood stroke associated with protein C or S deficiency and primary antiphospholipid syndrome. *Pediatric Neurology*, **9**, 67–70.

Dewitt, L.D. (1995) Antiphospholipid antibody syndrome. *In:* Bogousslavsky, J., Caplan, L (Eds) *Stroke Syndromes*. Cambridge: Cambridge University Press, p. 412–421.

Drillien, C.M. (1972) Abnormal neurologic signs in the first year of life in low-birthweight infants: possible prognostic significance. *Developmental Medicine and Child Neurology*, **14**, 573–584.

Flodmark, O., Lupton, B., Li, D., Stimac, G., Roland, E., Hill, A., Whitfield, M., Norman, M. (1989) MR imaging of periventricular leukomalacia in childhood. *American Journal of Radiology*, **152**, 583–590.

Göbel, U. (1994) Inherited or acquired disorders of blood coagulation in children with neurovascular complications. *Neuropediatrics*, **25**, 4–7.

Guzzetta, F., Shackelford, G., Volpe, S., Perlman, J., Volpe, J. (1986) Periventricular intraparenchymal echodensities in the premature newborn: Critical determinant of neurological outcome. *Pediatrics*, **78**, 995–1006.

Hagberg, B. (1979) Epidemiological and preventive aspects of cerebral palsy and severe mental retardation in Sweden. *European Journal of Pediatrics*, **130**, 71–78.

— Hagberg, G., Olow, I., von Wendt, L. (1989) The changing panorama of cerebral palsy in Sweden. *Acta Paediatrica Scandinavica*, **78**, 283–290.

Keeney, S.E., Adcock, E.W., McArdle, C.B. (1991) Prospective observations of 100 high-risk neonates by high-field (1.5 Tesla) magnetic resonance imaging of the central nervous system. II: Lesions associated with hypoxic-ischemic encephalopathy. *Pediatrics*, **87**, 431–438.

Khaw, C.W., Tidemann, A.J., Stern, L.M. (1994) Study of hemiplegic cerebral palsy with a review of the literature. *Journal of Paediatrics and Child Health*, **30**, 224–229.

Koch B, Braillier D, Eng G, Binder H. (1980) Computerized tomography in cerebral-palsied children. *Developmental Medicine and Child Neurology*, **22**, 595–607.

Koeda, T., Suganuma, I., Kohno, Y., Takamatsu, T., Takeshita, K. (1990) MR imaging of spastic diplegia. *Neuroradiology*, **32**, 187–190.

Konishi, Y., Kuriyama, M., Hayakawa, K., Konishi, K., Yasujima, M., Fujii, Y., Sudo, M., Ishii Y. (1990) Periventricular hyperintensity detected by magnetic resonance imaging in infancy. *Pediatric Neurology*, **6**, 229–232.

Korte, W., Otremba, H., Lutz, S., Flury, R., Schmid, L., Weissert, M. (1994) Childhood stroke at three years of age with transient protein C deficiency, familial antiphospholipid antibodies and F. XII deficiency - a family study. *Neuropediatrics*, **25**, 290–294.

Kotlarek, F., Rodewig, R., Brüll, D., Zeumer, H. (1981) Computed tomographic findings in congenital hemiparesis in childhood and their relation to etiology and prognosis. *Neuropediatrics*, **12**, 101–109.

Krägeloh-Mann, I., Hagberg, B., Petersen, D., Riethmüller, J., Gut, E., Michaelis, R. (1992) Bilateral spastic cerebral palsy - pathogenetic aspects from MRI. *Neuropediatrics*, **23**, 46–48.

— Petersen, D., Hagberg, B., Michaelis, R. (1994) Magnetic resonance imaging in the timing of pathological events - a study in bilateral spastic cerebral palsy children. *In:* Lou, H.C., Greisen, G., Falck Larsen, J. (Eds) *Brain Lesions in the Newborn. Alfred Benzon Symposium 37*, Copenhagen: Munksgaard Press, p. 178–191.

— — Hagberg, G., Vollmer, B., Hagberg, B., Michaelis, R. (1995) Bilateral spastic cerebral palsy - MRI pathology and origin. Analysis from a representative series of 56 cases. *Developmental Medicine and Child Neurology*, **37**, 379–397.

Lipper, M.H., Chason, D.P., Cail, W.S., Ferguson, R.D., Park, T.S., Phillips, L.H. (1991) MRI in cerebral palsy: correlation between clinical and MR findings. *Neuroradiology*, **33(Suppl)**, 618–620.

Mantovani J, Gerber G. (1984) 'Idiopathic' neonatal cerebral infarction. *AJDC*, **138**, 359–362.

Michaelis R, Rooschüz B, Dopfer R. (1980) Prenatal origin of congenital spastic hemiparesis. *Early Human Development*, **4**, 243–255.

50

— Asenbauer, C., Buchwald-Saal, M., Haas, G., Krägeloh-Mann, I. (1993) Transitory neurological findings in a population of at risk infants. *Early Human Development* **34:** 143–153.

— Niemann, G. (1995) *Entwicklungsneurologie und Neuropädiatrie - Grundlagen und diagnostische Strategien.* Stuttgart: Hippokrates.

Molteni, B., Oleari, G., Fedrizzi, E., Bracchi, M. (1987) Relation between CT patterns, clinical findings and etiological factors in children born at term, affected by congenital hemiparesis. *Neuropediatrics,* **18,** 75–80.

Mutch, L., Alberman, E., Hagberg, B., Kodama, K., Velickovic-Perat, M. (1992) Cerebral palsy epidemiology: where are we now and where are we going? *Developmental Medicine and Child Neurology,* **34,** 547–551.

Nelson, K., Ellenberg, J. (1982) Children who 'outgrew' cerebral palsy. *Pediatrics,* **69,** 529–536.

Niemann, G., Wakat, J.P., Krägeloh-Mann, I., Grodd, W., Michaelis, R. (1994) Congenital hemiparesis and periventricular leukomalacia: Pathogenetic aspects on magnetic resonance imaging. *Developmental Medicine and Child Neurology,* **36,** 943–950.

— Grodd, W., Schöning, M. (1996) Late remission of congenital hemiparesis: The value of MRI. *Neuropediatrics,* **27,** 197–201.

Pharoah, P., Cooke, T., Cooke, R., Rosenbloom, L. (1990) Birthweight specific trends in cerebral palsy. *Acrchives of Diseases in Childhood,* **65,** 602–606.

Piper, M.C., Mazer, B., Silver, K.M., Ramsay, M. (1988) Resolution of neurological symptoms in high-risk infants during the first two years of life. *Developmental Medicine and Child Neurology,* **30,** 26–35.

Rademaker, K.J., Groenendaal, F., Jansen, G.H., Eken, P., de Vries, L.S. (1994) Unilateral haemorrhagic parenchymal lesions in the preterm infant: shape, site and prognosis. *Acta Paediatrica,* **83,** 602–608.

Ravelli, A., Martini, A., Burgio, G.R. (1994) Antiphospholipid antibodies in paediatrics. *European Journal of Pediatrics,* **153,** 472–479.

Scher, M., Belfar, H., Martin, J., Painter, M. (1991) Destructive brain lesions of presumed fetal onset: antepartum causes of cerebral palsy. *Pediatrics,* **88,** 898–906.

Schöning, M., Staab, M., Walter, J., Niemann, G. (1993) Transcranial color duplex sonography in childhood and adolescence. Age dependence of flow velocities and waveform parameters. *Stroke ,* **24:** 1305–1309.

— Klein, R., Krägloh-Mann, I., Falck, M., Bien, S., Berg, P.A., Michaelis, R. (1994) Antiphospholipid antibodies in cerebrovascular ischemia and stroke in childhood. *Neuropediatrics,* **25,** 8–14.

Silver, R., MacGregor, S., Pasternak, J., Neely, S. (1992) Fetal stroke associated with elevated maternal anti-cardiolipin antibodies. *Obstetrics and Gynecology,* **80,** 497–499.

Stanley, F., Watson, L. (1992) Trends in perinatal mortality and cerebral palsy in Western Australia 1967 to 1985. *British Medical Journal,* **304,** 1658–1663.

Steinlin, M., Good, M., Martin, E., Bänziger, O., Largo, R.H., Boltshauser, E. (1993) Congenital hemiplegia: Morphology of cerebral lesions and pathogenetic aspects from MRI. *Neuropediatrics,* **24,** 224–229.

Süssová, J., Seidl, Z., Faber, J. (1990) Hemiparetic forms of cerebral palsy in relation to epilepsy and mental retardation. *Developmental Medicine and Child Neurology,* **32,** 792–795.

Takanashi, J., Sugita, K., Fujii, K., Niimi, H. (1995) Periventricular haemosiderin deposition in patients with congenital hemiplegia. *Developmental Medicine and Child Neurology,***37,** 1016–1019.

Takashima, S., Mito, T., Ando, Y. (1986) Pathogenesis of periventricular white matter hemorrhages in preterm infants. *Brain Development,* **8,** 25–30.

Taudorf, K., Hansen, F.J., Melchior, J.C., Pedersen, H. (1986) Spontaneous remission of cerebral palsy. *Neuropediatrics ,* **17,** 19–22.

Truwit, C.J., Barkovich, A.J., Koch, Th.K., Ferriero, D.M. (1992) Cerebral palsy: MR findings in 40 patients. *American Jouranl of Neuroradiology,* **13,** 67–78.

Uvebrant, P. (1988) Hemiplegic cerebral palsy - aetiology and outcome. *Acta Paediatrica Scandinavica,* **345 (suppl):** 1–100.

van Bogaert, P., Baleriaux, D., Christophe, C., Szliwowski, H.B. (1992) MRI of patients with cerebral palsy and normal CT scan. *Neuroradiology,* **34,** 52–56.

Vargha-Khadem, F., Isaacs, E., voan der Werf, S., Roob, S., Wilson, J. (1992) Development of intelligence and memory in children with hemiplegic cerebral palsy. The deleterious consequences of early seizures. *Brain ,***115,** 315–329.

Volpe, J.J. (1989a) Intraventricular haemorrhage in the premature infant - current concepts. Part II. *Annals of Neurology,* **25,** 109–116.

— (1989b) Current concepts of brain injury in the premature infant. *American Journal of Radiology,* **153,** 243–251.

— (1995) *Neurology of the Newborn. 3rd edn.* Philadelphia: W.B. Saunders.

— (1996a) Subplate neurons - missing link in brain injury of the premature infant? *Pediatrics,* **97,** 112–113.

— (1996b) Brain injury in the premature infant: current concepts. *Biology of the Newborn,* **69,** 167–169.

Wiklund, L.M., Uvebrant, P., Flodmark, O. (1990) Morphology of cerebral lesions in children with congenital hemiplegia. A study with computed tomography. *Neuroradiology,* **32,** 179–186.

— — (1991) Hemiplegic cerebral palsy: correlation between CT morphology and clinical findings. *Developmental Medicine and Child Neurology,* **33,** 512–523.

World Health Organization. (1980) *International Classification of Impairments, Disabilities and Handicap.* Geneva: WHO.

Yokochi, K., Aiba, K., Horie, M., Inukai, K., Fujimoto, S., Kodama, M., Kodama, K. (1991) Magnetic resonance imaging in children with spastic diplegia: Correlation with the severity of their motor and mental abnormality. *Developmental Medicine and Child Neurology* , **33,** 18–25.

5
CLINICAL PRESENTATION
AND NEUROLOGY

Paul Uvebrant

Congenital hemiplegia occurs in about five per 10 000 live births (Hagberg et al. 1975a, b, 1996; Dale and Stanley 1980). Somewhat higher figures, of six to seven per 10 000, have been reported from Sweden and Western Australia (Uvebrant 1988, Hagberg et al. 1989, Stanley and Watson 1992), but lower, about four per 10 000, from England and Ireland (Dowding and Barry 1988, Goodman and Yude 1996). It is not known whether this reflects real differences between the countries or differences in case finding and reporting systems. For purposes of clinical studies, however, Goodman and Yude (1996) found that some incompleteness in ascertainment and recruitment did not significantly affect the representativeness of samples of congenital hemiplegia.

The distribution of congenital hemiplegia by gestational age can be seen in Table 5.1. Three of four children with congenital hemiplegia are born at term, to be compared to one-third in spastic diplegia (Hagberg et al. 1996). Males are more often affected than females with a rate of about 1.4:1 (Perlstein and Hood 1954, Goutieres et al. 1972, Uvebrant 1988) and right-sided hemiplegia is more common than left-sided – 56% of almost 1 500 subjects had a right-sided hemiplegia (Stewart 1948, Perlstein and Hood 1954, Crothers and Paine 1959, Ingram 1964, Churchill 1968, Goutieres et al. 1972, Glenting 1976, Uvebrant 1988). The cause of this preponderance of left-hemisphere lesions is unknown. A hypothesis that the dominant hemisphere should be more vulnerable to early damage than the non-dominant was contradicted by the finding of Goodman (1994) that children with a family history of left-handedness were disproprtionately more likely to have a right rather than a left hemiplegia. Overall, there are no major differences in disability or additional impairments between people with congenital right and left hemiplegia (Khaw et al. 1994).

Early manifestations of congenital hemiplegia
"Abnormality of movements in congenital hemiplegia will first become obvious at a time when it normally begins to be controlled by the cerebral cortex" according to Tizard (1961, p. 30). The signs of hemiplegia rarely present in the young infant but develop gradually during the second half of the first year. This silent period has repeatedly been noted (Lyon 1961, Goutières et al. 1972) and was verified by Bouza and colleagues (1994) in the careful follow up of term infants with unilateral brain lesions documented by ultrasound and MRI in the neonatal period. Stewart (1948) showed that weakness and hypotonia are the indicators of hemiplegia in early infancy and consequently its cerebral nature may escape recognition.

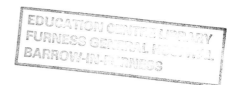

TABLE 5.1
Distribution of congenital hemiplegia by gestational age groups.
Birth years 1975–1990.
(Hagberg et al. 1996).

Gestational age (wk)	n	%
<28	8	3
28–31	12	5
32–36	39	16
>36	179	75
Total	238	100

However, even such early signs of hypotonia and weakness were negated by Bouza and colleagues (1994). Yokochi and coworkers (1995) retrospectively studied videorecordings from children with hemiplegia aged from 2 to 8 months. At 7 to 8 months they could support their weight on the flexed arm on the affected side in the prone position but in the supine, only half of the infants could fully extend the knee. They had deficient forward movement of the arm and deficient opening of the hand.

The mean age at diagnosis of congenital hemiplegia in a retrospective study of 148 children was 12 months, 3 months after the parents first seriously suspected something was wrong (Uvebrant 1988). A first peak age for diagnosis was found at 3 to 6 months when grasping was expected to develop, early handedness was a strong predictor of hemiplegia with two-thirds of the children being left- or right-handed before 12 months of age (Cohen and Duffner 1981), with a mean age at lateralisation of 6 months (Uvebrant 1988). The earlier the handedness, the more severe the hemiplegia.

A second peak age for diagnosis was during the second year of life when the child began to walk. Unsupported walking was achieved by half of the children by 18 months of age, which is slightly delayed when compared with normally developing children. This was true also when children born preterm and children with learning disabilities were excluded. As stated by David Scrutton in chapter 6 of this book, all children with congenital hemiplegia will eventually learn to walk, unless there is also a severe general developmental disorder or profound intractable epilepsy. This is illustrated in Table 5.2. Almost half of the children will not crawl on their hands and knees in an ordinary way, but shuffle on their bottom, tummy or in some individual way.

In some infants deterioration with loss of preexisting skills can be observed (Bouza et al. 1994). Yet the opposite may also be the case – Niemann and colleagues (1996) described late remission of congenital hemiplegia with disappearance of symptoms between the ages of 3 and 10 years.

Severity of the motor and sensory impairment
About one of five children with congenital hemiplegia has a severe motor impairment, half of them have a moderate, and one-third a mild impairment (Ingram 1964, Goutières et al.

TABLE 5.2
Early development in children with congenital hemiplegia
(Uvebrant 1988).

Sitting
   Delayed in 22% of normally gifted children
     and 74% of children with learning disabilities

Prewalking locomotion
   Only 43% crawled on hands and knees

Walking
   Mean   17 mo
   50%   <18 mo (normal 97%)
   23%   18–21 mo
   22%   >21 mo

Handedness
   Mean   6 mo
   66%   <12 mo (early)
   31%   12 mo–3 y (normal)
   3%   >3 y (late)

1972, Claeys et al. 1983, Uvebrant 1988). The impairment dominates in the arm and hand in about half of the children, in the lower limb in a third, and affects the upper and lower limb equally in one-fifth (Goutieres et al. 1972, Rooschuz 1976, Bertelsmeier 1981, Uvebrant 1988). Arm-dominated hemiplegia is most common in children born at term, whereas the leg is more often more impaired in children born preterm. Table 5.3 shows the distribution of level of motor and sensory impairment.

THE ARM
Proximal power is preserved in the upper limb (Brown et al. 1987) and the mechanical restriction of movements increases towards the periphery (Stewart 1948), with restricted extension of the elbow in about one half (Uvebrant 1988).

The most difficult movements are supinating the forearm, followed by pronation and, according to Yokochi and coworkers (1992) flexing the shoulder. Apart from the functional effects of a pronated hand, the radial head may be subluxated and further restrict elbow extension (Pletcher et al. 1976).

THE HAND
A major difficulty for individuals with hemiplegia is the flexed wrist, or 'drop hand'. When asked about actual hand function (Uvebrant 1988), about one-third of subjects considered it to be good, one-third moderately impaired (a good helper) and one-third poor. Of the latter, two-thirds used their hand as support whereas one-third considered the hand completely useless.

The sensory function of the hand is impaired in about half of children with hemiplegia (Uvebrant 1988). Discriminatory faculties such as stereognosis and graphaesthesia are more often affected than modalities such as pain, touch and temperature which are usually normal. Van Heest and

TABLE 5.3
Motor and sensory impairments in congenital hemiplegia (Uvebrant 1988).

	Good	Moderately impaired	Poor
	%	%	%
Gait	60	30	10
Hand function			
Motor	50	40	10
Stereognosis	50	30	20
Resulting function	⅓	⅓	⅓

colleagues (1993) found sensibility deficiencies, even proprioception deficits, to be very common and the rule rather than the exception and Cooper and coworkers (1995) stressed the importance of identifying these often-overlooked impairments in order to maximise the functional potential of the children. Impairment of hand function is closely related to the quality of sensitivity (Feldkamp et al. 1985).

According to Brown and colleagues (1987), poor hand function correlates also with the loss of both power and speed of movement in the affected hand. Grasping is not only hampered by the motor and discriminatory impairments but also by impaired tactile and anticipatory control (Eliasson et al. 1995). Although children with hemiplegia may have disturbed sensory feedback, their main disability stems from impaired central coordination of motor activity (Eliasson et al. 1992).

Farmer and coworkers (1991) studied the plasticity of central motor pathways in children with hemiplegic cerebral palsy (CP) and Carr and colleagues (1993) suggested reorganisation with ipsilateral motor pathways from the undamaged motor cortex to the hemiplegic hand by corticospinal axons branching abnormally and projecting bilaterally to homologous motor-neurone pools on both sides of the spinal cord. Hand function is further discussed by Walsh and Brown in chapter 9 of this book.

THE LEG

In the lower limb there may be restriction of external rotation in the hip and also difficulties in rotating the hip internally (Yokochi et al. 1992). Some degree of hamstring contracture may be present. However, this rarely constitutes a significant problem and is found in less than one of five individuals with hemiplegia (Uvebrant 1988). A spastic quadriceps (Csongradi et al. 1979) and a poor regulation of ankle plantarflexion power may result in hyperextension of the knee (Simon et al. 1978).

THE FOOT

Active dorsiflexion of the ankle is the most difficult movement in the leg. The peripheral and central mechanisms of hind foot equinus in hemiplegia have been discussed by Lin and coworkers (1992) who state that gait equinus cannot be explained merely in terms of central paralytic foot-drop. A developmental mechanism needs to be involved. Apart from the equinus position, a varus deformity of the foot is somewhat more common than valgus (Bennet et al. 1982).

GAIT

In a study by Uvebrant (1988), a mild disturbance or a near-normal walking pattern was present in about 60%, a moderate limp in 30% and severe lameness in 10% of the children. Hyperextension of the knee was noted in about a quarter and the typical circumduction seen in adult-onset hemiplegia was only seen in 1 of 10 people. A normal heel strike was present in one of five whereas about 40% each had a foot-flat gait or a toe strike on the hemiplegic side.

Although the lower limb is the more often affected among children born preterm, the severity of impairment of walking is inversely correlated to gestational age. A severe impairment is twice as common among children born at term compared with preterm born children with congenital hemiplegia.

There are complex patterns of motor impairments in the lower extremity and several gait patterns can be recognised (Winters et al. 1987). A subclassification of congenital hemiplegia based on gait patterns may be useful for treatment purposes – see chapters 7 and 8 in this book. More information on physical assessment and aims of treatment is also given in chapter 6.

THE FACE

There is a relative sparing of facial movements in prenatal-onset hemiparesis (Lenn and Freinkel 1989) that has been attributed to neural plasticity (Lenn and Thurston 1983). Still about one-third of individuals with hemiparesis have some asymmetry of the face at rest and when voluntary or emotional movements are added, a majority have discernible unilateral weakness (Freud 1891, Stewart 1948, Ingram 1964, Uvebrant 1988).

The sparing of the face and the rarity of dysarthria (see below), as well as the paucity of other bulbar signs in congenital hemiplegia may not only be due to neural plasticity, but also to bilateral control of bulbar functions.

Neurological findings

MUSCULAR TONE

An initial phase of decreased tone may be present in the infant and young child with congenital hemiplegia (Stewart 1948). Thereafter, hypertonia is almost uniformly present. Refined methods to detect and quantify spasticity have been developed and will be important to further subclassify congenital hemiplegia, for better understanding of pathophysiology and evaluation of treatment (Sloan et al. 1992; Lin et al. 1994a, b). The extent of affected muscle tone and tendon reflexes is listed in Table 5.4.

TENDON REFLEXES

Hyperactive tendon reflexes are invariably present but may be attenuated by contractures and orthopaedic surgery (Ingram 1964). As may be expected, neurological signs are often not strictly unilateral. Children born preterm are particularly prone to hyperactive reflexes or a positive Babinski sign in the contralateral leg and foot. Sometimes it may be difficult to separate hemiplegia from diplegia, but as long as the impairment on the 'normal' side is not associated with any degree of disability, the diagnosis should be hemiplegia.

TABLE 5.4.
Neurological signs in congenital hemiplegia. Muscle tone and tendon reflexes.
(Uvebrant 1988).

	Born preterm %	Born at term %
Arm		
Increased tone	56	69
Hyperactive tendon reflexes	56	74
Leg		
Increased tone	81	73
Hyperactive quadriceps reflex	97	85
Hyperactive achilles reflex	75	64
Babinski sign	81	75
Bilateral signs	56	39

NEUROLOGICAL SIGNS

Dyskinetic signs sometimes appear at a later age, mainly in the form of athetoid hand movements (Ingram 1964, Goutieres et al. 1972) or more rarely in dystonic posturing (Hagberg, unpublished data), signs which may progress over the years (Dooling and Adams 1975). As Table 5.5 shows, signs of ataxia such as tremor and dysmetria are rarely seen (in less than 10% of people with hemiplegia).

Growth

General growth, such as height and weight, is not impaired in congenital hemiplegia (Maekava et al. 1979). Head circumference is most often close to normal, if a small subgroup (10 to 15%) of children with learning disability with reduced head size or hemiatrophy of the skull are excluded.

Undergrowth of the hemiplegic side is an enigmatic phenomenon. Several explanations have been suggested (Stevenson et al. 1995). Holt (1961) and Tachdjian and Minear (1958) proposed disuse, Wilkins (1955) decreased blood flow and Penfield and Robertson (1943) lesions of the postcentral cortex.

The severity of undergrowth correlates to severity of motor and stereognostic impairment, but it is not a direct correlation. There are several examples of severe undergrowth of functionally preserved extremities, as well as the opposite.

Shortening of the arm is more pronounced than that of the leg in most cases, it may be more embarrassing than the actual palsy (Ingram 1964). Not only the arm and leg are undergrown, but also fingers and nails on the affected side. Dwarfing of the extremity is very frequent but seldom severe, most often just 1 or 2 centimetres. Feldkamp and colleagues (1985) found no further increase in the differences in leg length after the age of 8 years. Vasomotor disturbance may also be present in the affected limbs.

TABLE 5.5.
Neurological signs in congenital hemiplegia (Uvebrant 1988).

A pure spastic syndrome	72%	
Dyskinetic signs	21%	(Term 23%, Preterm 13%)
Ataxia	7%	
Facial weakness	31%	(Term 36%, Preterm 13%)

Scoliosis

Contrary to what may be expected, the incidence of scoliosis is low in congenital hemiplegia. Between 10 and 20% are affected, most often in a mild way (Horstmann and Boyer 1982, Uvebrant 1988). However, a majority have some asymmetries of the shoulders, often with atrophy and a slightly elevated shoulder. There may also be a curvature of the spine due to shortening of the leg.

The rarity of scoliosis in congenital hemiplegia indicates that factors other than asymmetry in muscular tone must be of crucial importance for the development of this deformity. Bleck (1975, 1987) suggested that impaired equilibrium reactions and postural control (Gregoric et al. 1981) may be more important than asymmetrical muscle tone, explaining why scoliosis is more common in ataxic CP (Rosenthal et al. 1974) and in non-ambulatory patients with CP (Samilson and Perry 1975). Another high-risk population for scoliosis is children with lower motor neurone impairments such as polyneuropathies (Hagberg et al. 1983). Lower motor neurone lesions are extremely rare in congenital hemiplegia, less than 5% have signs of such lesions (Ingram 1964, Uvebrant 1988).

Additional impairments

LEARNING DISABILITY

Learning disability accompanies the hemiplegia in about one of five individuals. The disability is severe in a minority, a quarter of those with learning disability (Saunders 1961 Goutières et al. 1972, Claeys et al. 1983, Uvebrant 1988). Severe learning disability affects mainly children born at term. Occasional reports have stated that right-sided hemiplegia is more often associated with learning disability (McIntire 1947, Woods 1961) but most studies have found no difference between right- and left-sided hemiplegia with regard to the occurrence of such disability.

As might be expected, the learning disability correlates with the severity of hemiplegia and also with the association of other additional neuroimpairments such as epilepsy (Perlstein and Hood 1955, Gibbs et al. 1963, Jabbour and Lundervold 1963, O'Reilly 1971, Goutières et al. 1972). Mental impairments are further discussed by Muter and Vargha-Khadem in chapter 13.

EPILEPSY

Epilepsy is, depending on how it is defined and on the population studied, present in a quarter to a third of individuals with hemiplegic CP (Asher and Schonell 1950, Perlstein and Hood

1954, Glenting 1963, Ingram 1964, Goutieres et al. 1972, Uvebrant 1988). Epilepsy and learning disability are the major accompanying impairments in congenital hemiplegia. They are discussed in detail in separate chapters in this book, as are cognitive, behavioural and emotional aspects.

VISION

Severe visual impairment is rare in congenital hemiplegia. Although less frequent than in other spastic or dyskinetic forms of CP (Ipata et al. 1994) abnormalities such as strabismus, impaired acuity, stereopsis or visual fields are common (Schenk-Rootlieb et al. 1992, Mercuri et al. 1996). Considering the close anatomical connection between the optic radiation and lateral ventricles, in particular the posterior and temporal horns, it seems plausible that visual tracts can be affected in hemiplegia with periventricular lesions, and such cases are numerous as indicated by CT (Wiklund and Uvebrant 1991) and by MRI scans (Nieman et al. 1994). The functional effects of such lesions in the retrochiasmatic parts of the visual systems are not fully known so far. Studies on cerebral visual disturbance in infantile encephalopathy, such as the one by van Neiuwenhuizen (1987), are needed to clarify the issue.

Children with shunt-treated hydrocephalus added to the hemiplegia seem to be at special risk for visual disturbances (Uvebrant 1988).

HEARING

Hearing is most often normal. A sensorineural hearing impairment may sometimes be found, especially in children born preterm. An association with hyperbilirubinaemia in the neonatal period has been discussed (for example, Thiringer 1998). More central auditory perceptual deficiencies have been shown by Hugdahl and Carlsson (1994).

SPEECH

Language development is well preserved in congenital hemiplegia, irrespective of whether the brain lesion is right or left sided (Feldkamp et al. 1985, Carlsson et al. 1994). Also speech disturbances (i.e. dysarthria) are rare (Van Mourik et al. 1994), it seems as if bilateral brain lesions are prerequisites for such impairments to occur in congenital CP (Uvebrant and Carlsson 1994). See also Chapter 13 in this book.

DISABILITY

Disability is the individuals' experience of her or his limitations to fulfil the role that is normal (depending on age, sex, and social and cultural factors) for that individual (World Health Organization 1980). The disability experienced depends not only on the severity of impairment, but also on the physical milieu and on attitudes.

When asked about disability, about 40% considered it negligible or mild, about the same proportion experienced a moderate and less than one of five had a severe disability (Uvebrant 1988).

In his study on the course and prognosis of congenital hemiplegia, Glenting (1963) found that "the prognosis for a certain handicap is unfavourably influenced by the presence of other handicaps" (p. 260). Such a tendency for impairments to interact and potentiate each other, not only in an additive but in a multiplying way was found also by Uvebrant (1988). In the population studied, the 16% of children with a severe disability contributed 63% of all severe impairments recorded. As previously stated by Hagberg (1978) "the multihandicap pattern presented itself as the dominating factor for serious neuropaediatric problems of persisting type" (p. 122).

REFERENCES

Asher, P., Schonell, F. (1950) A survey of 400 cases of cerebral palsy in childhood. *Archives of Diseases in Children,* **25,** 360–379.

Bennet, G.C., Rang, M., Jones, D. (1982) Varus and valgus deformities of the foot in cerebral palsy. *Developmental Medicine and Child Neuroogy,* **24,** 499–503.

Bertelsmeier, S. (1981) *Klinische und elektroenzephalographische Untersuchungen bei Kindern mit ange-borener spastischer Hemiparese und cerebrale Anfällen.* Inaugural PhD Dissertation. Tübingen: H Vogler.

Bleck, E.E. (1975) Deformities of the spine and pelvis in cerebral palsy. *In:* Samilson (Ed.) *Orthopaedic Aspects of Cerebral Palsy.Clinics in Developmental Medicine, Nos 52/53.* London: Mac Keith Press, pp. 124–144.

— (1987) *Orthopaedic Management in Cerebral Palsy.Clinics in Developmental Medicine, Nos 99/100.* London: Mac Keith Press.

Bouza, H., Rutherford, M., Acolet, D., Pennock, J.M., Dubowitz, L.M. (1994) Evolution of early hemiplegic signs in full-term infants with unilateral brain lesions in the neonatal period: a prospective study. *Neuropediatrics,* **25,** 201–207.

Brown, J.K., van Rensburg, F., Walsh, G., Lakie, M., Wright, G.W. (1987) A neurological study of hand function of hemiplegic children. *Developmental Medicine and Child Neurology,* **29,** 287–304.

Carlsson, G., Uvebrant, P., Hugdahl, K., Arvidsson, J., Wiklund, L.M., von Wendt, L. (1994) Verbal and non-verbal function of children with right- versus left-hemiplegic cerebral palsy of pre- and perinatal origin. *Developmental Medicine and Child Neurology,* **36,** 503–512.

Carr, L.J., Harrison, L.M., Evans, A.L., Stephens, J.A. (1993) Patterns of central motor reorganization in hemi-plegic cerebral palsy. *Brain,* **116,** 1223–47.

Churchill, J.A. (1968) A study of hemiplegic cerebral palsy *Developmental Medicine and Child Neurology,* 10, 453–459.

Claeys, V., Deonna, T., Chrzannowski, R. (1983) Congenital hemiparesis: the spectrum of lesions. A clinical and computerized tomographic study of 37 cases. *Helvetica Paediatrica Acta,* **38,** 439–455.

Cohen, J., Duffner, P. (1981) Prognostic indicators in hemiparetic cerebral palsy. *Annals of Neurology,* **9,** 353–357.

Cooper, J., Majnemer, A., Rosenblatt, B., Birnbaum, R. (1995) The determination of sensory deficits in children with hemiplegic cerebral palsy. *Journal of Child Neurology,* **10,** 300–309.

Crothers, B., Paine, R.S. (1959) The Natural History of Cerebral Palsy. Oxford: Oxford University Press, p. 91.

Csongradi, J., Bleck, E. E., Ford, W. F. (1979) Gait electromyography in normal and spastic children with special reference to the quadriceps femoris and hamstring muscles. *Developmental Medicine and Child Neurology,* **21,** 738–84.

Dale, A., Stanley, F.J. (1980) An epidemiological study of cerebral palsy in Western Australia, 1956-1975. II. Spastic cerebral palsy and perinatal factors. *Developmental Medicine and Child Neurology,* **22,** 13–25.

Dooling, E., Adams, R. (1975) The pathological anatomy of post-hemiplegic athetosis. *Brain,* **98,** 29–48.

Dowding, V. M., Barry, C. (1988) Cerebral palsy: changing patterns of birthweight and gestational age (1967/81). *Irish Medical Journal,* **81,** 24–29.

Eliasson, A.C., Gordon, A.M., Forssberg, H. (1992) Impaired anticipatory control of isometric forces during grasping by children with cerebral palsy. *Developmental Medicine and Child Neurology,* **34,** 216–225.

— — — (1995) Tactile control of isometric fingertip forces during grasping in children with cerebral palsy. *Developmental Medicine and Child Neurology,* **37,** 72–84.

Farmer, S.F., Harrison, L.M., Ingram, D.A., Stephens, J.A. (1991) Plasticity of central motor pathways in children with hemiplegic cerebral palsy. *Neurology,* **41,** 1505–1510.

Feldkamp, M., Schuknecht, C., Eisenkolb, T. (1985) Accompanying symptoms in infantile spastic hemiplegia. *Zeitschrift für Orthopädie,* **123,** 300–305.

61

Freud, S., Rie, O. (1891) *Klinische Studie über die halbseitige Cerebralhämung der Kinder.* Vienna: Moritz Perles.

Gibbs, F., Gibbs, E., Meyer, A., Perlstein, M., Rich, C. (1963) Electroencephalographic and clinical aspects of cerebral palsy. *Pediatrics,* **32,** 73.

Glenting, P. (1963) Course and prognosis of congenital spastic hemiplegia. *Developmental Medicine and Child Neurology,* **5,** 252–60.

— (1976) Variations in the population of congenital (pre- and perinatal) cases of cerebral palsy in Danish counties east of the Little Belt during the years 1950-1969. *Ugeskrift for Laeger,* **138,** 2984–2991.

Goodman, R. (1994) Childhood hemiplegia: is the side of lesion influenced by a family history of left-handedness? *Developmental Medicine and Child Neurology,* **36,** 406–411.

— Yude, C. (1996) Do incomplete ascertainment and recruitment matter? – a study in childhood hemiplegia. *Developmental Medicine and Child Neurology,* **38,** 156–165.

Goutières, F., Challamel, M-J., Aicardi, J., Gilly, R. (1972) Les hempilegies congenitales. Semiologie, etiologie et pronostic. *Archives Francaises de Pediatrie,* **29,** 839–851.

Gregoric, M., Pecac, F., Trontelj, J.V., Dimitrijevic, M.R. (1981) Postural control in scoliosis. *Acta Orthopedica Scandinavica,* **52,** 59–63.

Hagberg, B. (1978) The epidemiological panorama of major neuropaediatric handicaps in Sweden. *In:* Apley, J. (Ed.) *Care of the Handicapped Child. Clinics in Developmental Medicine, No. 67.* London: Mac Keith Press, p.111–124.

— Hagberg, G., Olow, I. (1975) The changing panorama of cerebral palsy in Sweden 1954-1970. I. Analysis of the general changes. *Acta Paediatrica Scandinavica,* **64,** 187–192.

——— (1975) The changing panorama of cerebral palsy in Sweden 1954-1970. II. Analysis of the various. syndromes. *Acta Paediatrica Scandinavica,* **64,** 193–200.

— Westerberg, B., Hagne, I., Sellden, U. (1983) Hereditary motor and sensory neuropathies in Swedish children. III. De- and remyelinating type in 10 sporadic cases. *Acta Paediatrica Scandinavica,* **72,** 537–544.

— Hagberg, G., Olow, I., von Wendt, L. (1989) The changing panorama of cerebral palsy in Sweden. V. The birth year period 1979-1982. *Acta Paediatrica Scandinavica,* **78,** 283–290.

———— (1996) The changing panorama of cerebral palsy in Sweden 1954-1970. VII. Prevalence and origin in the birth year period 1987-90. *Acta Paediatrica,* **85,** 954–960.

Holt, K. (1961) Growth disturbance. In: Bax, M. (Ed.) *Hemiplegic Cerebral Palsy in Children and Adults, Clinics in Developmental Medicine, No. 4.* London: Mac Keith Press, p. 39–53.

Horstmann, H., Boyer, B. (1982) The incidence of scoliosis in cerebral palsy. American Academy for Cerebral Palsy and Developmental Medicine meeting 1981. *Developmental Medicine and Child Neurology,* **24,** 235. (Abstract).

Hugdahl, K., Carlsson, G. (1994) Dichotic listening and focused attention in children with hemiplegic cerebral palsy. *Journal of Clinical and Experimental Neuropsychology,* **16,** 84–92.

Ingram, T. (1964) *Paediatric Aspects of Cerebral Palsy.* London: Livingstone.

Ipata, A.E., Cioni, G., Bottai, P., Fazzi, B., Canapicchi, R., Van Hof-Van Duin, J. (1994) Acuity card testing in children with cerebral palsy related to magnetic resonance images, mental levels and motor abilities. *Brain and Development,* **16,** 195–203.

Jabbour, J., Lundervold, A. (1963) Hemiplegia: A clinical and electroencephalographic study in childhood. *Developmental Medicine and Child Neurology,* **5,** 24–31.

Khaw, C.W., Tidemann, A.J., Stern, L.M. (1994) Study of hemiplegic cerebral palsy with a review of the literature. *Journal of Paediatric Child Health,* **30,** 224–229.

Lenn, N.J., Freinkel, A.J. (1989) Facial sparing as a feature of prenatal-onset hemiparesis. *Pediatric Neurology,* **5,** 291–295.

— Thurston, S.E. (1983) Is facial sparing in children with prenatal hemiparesis evidence for neural plasticity? *Annals of Neurology,* **14,** 371. (Abstract).

Lin, J.P., Brown, J.K. (1992) Peripheral and central mechanisms of hindfoot equinus in childhood hemiplegia. *Developmental Medicine and Child Neurology,* **34,** 949–965.

—— Brotherstone, R. (1994a) Assessment of spasticity in hemiplegic cerebral palsy. I. Proximal lower-limb reflex excitability. *Developmental Medicine and Child Neurology,* **36,** 116–129.

——— (1994b) Assessment of spasticity in hemiplegic cerebral palsy. II: Distal lower-limb reflex excitability and function. *Developmental Medicine and Child Neurology,* **36,** 290–303.

Lyon, G. (1961) First signs and mode of onset of congenital hemiplegia. In: Bax, M. (Ed.) *Hemiplegic Cerebral Palsy in Children and Adults, Clinics in Developmental Medicine, No. 4.* London: Mac Keith Press, p. 33–38.

McIntire, T. (1947) A study of the distribution of physical handicap and mental diagnosis in cerebral palsied children. *American Journal of Mental Deficiency,* **51,** 624–626.

Maekava, K., Ochiai, Y., Kokubun, Y., Tsuzura, S., Yamazaki, Y. (1979) Physical growth of cerebral palsy of different clinical types. Forty-two cases of cerebral palsy diagnosed before age of twelve months. *Jikeikai Medical Journal,* **26,** 77–83.

Mercuri, E., Spano, M., Bruccini, G., Frisone, M.F., Trombetta, J.C., Blandino, A., Longo, M., Guzzetta, F. (1996) Visual outcome in children with congenital hemiplegia: Correlation with MRI findings. *Neuropediatrics,* **27,** 184–8.

Minear, Niemann, G., Wakat, J.P., Krägeloh-Mann, I., Grodd, W., Michaelis, M. (1994) Congenital hemiparesis and periventricular leukomalacia: Pathogenetic aspects on magnetic resonance imaging. *Developmental Medicine and Child Neurology,* **36,** 943–950.

Nieman, G., Grodd, W., Schöning, M. (1996) Late remission of congenital hemiparesis: The value of MRI. *Neuropediatrics,* **27,** 197–201.

O'Reilly, D. (1971) The future of the cerebral palsied child. *Developmental Medicine and Child Neurology,* **13,** 635–640.

Penfield, W., Robertson, J.S.M. (1943) Growth asymmetry due to lesions of the post central cerebral cortex. *Archives of Neurology and Psychiatry,* **50,** 405–430.

Perlstein, M.G., Hood, P.N. (1954) Infantile spastic hemiplegia. I. Incidence. *Pediatrics,* **14,** 436–441.

— — (1955) Infantile pastic hemiplegia III. Intelligence. *Pediatrics,* **15,** 676–682.

Pletcher, D. F-J., Hoffer, M.M., Koffman, D.M. (1976) Non-traumatic dislocation of the radial head in cerebral palsy. *Journal of Bone and Joint Surgery,* **58A,** 104–105.

Rooschuz, B. (1976) *Klinische Untersuchungen zum Krankheitsbild der angeborenen spastischen Hemiparese.* Inaugural PhD Dissertation. Tübingen, Germany: B v Sprangenberg KG.

Rosenthal, R., Levine, D., McCarver, C. (1974) The occurrence of scoliosis in cerebral palsy. *Developmental Medicine and Child Neurology,* **16,** 664–667.

Samilson, R.L., Perry, J. (1975) The orthopaedic assessment in cerebral palsy. *In:* Samilson, R.L. (Ed.) *Orthopaedic Aspects of Cerebral Palsy.Clinics in Developmental Medicine, Nos 52/53.* London: Mac Keith Press. p. 35–70.

Saunders, R. (1961) Studies on intelligence in hemiplegic children. In: Bax, M. (Ed.) *Hemiplegic Cerebral Palsy in Children and Adults, Clinics in Developmental Medicine, No. 4.* London: Mac Keith Press, p. 67–70.

Schenk-Rootlieb, A.J.F., van Nieuwenhuisen, O., van der Graaf, Y., Wittebol-Post, D., Willemse, J. (1992) The prevalence of cerebral visual disturbance in children with cerebral palsy. *Developmental Medicine and Child Neurology,* **34,** 473–480.

Simon, S. R., Deutsch, S.D., Nuzzo, R.M., Mansour, M.J., Jackson, J.L.K., Koskinen, M., Rosenthal, R.K. (1978) Genu recurvatum in spastic cerebral palsy. *Journal of Bone and Joint Surgery,* **60A,** 882–894.

Sloan, R.L., Sinclair, E., Thompson, J., Taylor, S., Pentland, B. (1992) Inter-rater reliability of the modified Ashworth Scale for spasticity in hemiplegic patients. *International Journal of Rehabilitation Research,* **15,** 158–161.

Stanley, F. J., Watson, L. (1992) Trends in perinatal mortality and cerebral palsy in Western Australia, 1967 to 1985. *Brittish Medical Journal,* **304,** 1658–1663.

Stewart, R. (1948) Infantile cerebral hemiplegia - clinical features and pathological anatomy. *Edinburgh Medical Journal,* **55,** 488–505.

Stevenson, R.D., Roberts, C.D., Vogtle, L. (1995) The effects of non-nutritional factors on growth in cerebral palsy. *Developmental Medicine and Child Neurology,* **37,** 124–130.

Süssova, J., Seidl, Z., Faber, J. (1990) Hemiparic forms of cerebral palsy in relation to epilepsy and mental retardation. *Developmental Medicine and Child Neurology,* **32,** 792–795.

Tachdjian, M., Minear, W. (1958) Sensory disturbances in the hands of children with cerebral palsy. *Journal of Bone and Joint Surgery,* **40A,** 85–90.

Thiringer, K. (1988) Disorders of hearing. *In:* Levene, M. J., Bennet, M. J., Punt, J. (Eds) *Fetal and Neonatal Neurology and Neurosurgery.* Edinburgh: Churchill Livingstone, p. 547–549.

Tizard, P. (1961) Observations on the early manifestations of infantile hemiplegia. In: Bax, M. (Ed.) *Hemiplegic Cerebral Palsy in Children and Adults, Clinics in Developmental Medicine, No. 4.* London: Mac Keith Press, pp. 30–32.

Uvebrant, P. (1988) Hemiplegic cerebral palsy. Aetiology and outcome. *Acta Paediatrica Scandinavica,* **Suppl 345,** 1-100.

— Carlsson, G. (1994) Speech in children with cerebral palsy. *Acta Paediatrica,* **83,** 779. (Commentary).

63

Van Heest, A., House, J., Putnam, M. (1993) Sensibility deficiencies in the hands of children with spastic hemiplegia. *Journal of Hand Surgery (Am)*, **18**, 278–281.

Van Mourik, M., Boon, P., Paquie, P., Lormans, A., Van Dongen, H. (1994) Speech characteristics in children with congenital hemiplegia. *Acta Paediatrica*, **83**, 317–318.

Van Nieuwenhuiszen, O. (1987) *Cerebral Disturbance in Infantile Encephalopathy*. Dordrecht, The Netherlands: Martinus Nijhoff.

Wiklund, L.M., Uvebrant, P. (1991) Hemiplegic cerebral palsy: correlation between CT morphology and clinical findings. *Developmental Medicine and Child Neurology*, **33**, 512–523.

Wilkins, L. (1955) Hormonal influences on growth. *Annals of New York Academy of Science*, **60**, 541–806.

Winters, T.F., Gage, J.R., Hicks, R. (1987) Gait patterns in spastic hemiplegia in children and young adults. *Journal of Bone and Joint Surgery*, **69-A**, 437–441.

Woods, G. (1961) Natural history of hemiplegia. *In:* Bax, M. (Ed.) *Hemiplegic Cerebral Palsy in Children and Adults, Clinics in Developmental Medicine, No. 4*. London: Mac Keith Press, p. 26–29.

World Health Organization. (1980) *International Classification of Impairments, Disabilities and Handicap*. Geneva: WHO.

Yokochi, K., Hosoe, A., Kodama, M., Kodama, K. (1992) Assessment of upper and lower extremity movements in hemiplegic children. *Brain and Development*, **14**, 18–22.

— Yokochi, M., Kodama, K. (1995) Motor function of infants with spastic hemiplegia. *Brain and Development*, **17**, 42–48.

6
PHYSICAL ASSESSMENT AND AIMS OF TREATMENT

David Scrutton

Writing about the assessment and treatment of a disorder with few proven treatments, a mixed aetiology, wide-ranging severity and additional problems is never going to be easy. There is nothing that can be written that does not risk the reader thinking, 'But what if…?' or 'But *I* can!' or 'I've never seen *that* happen'. For this reason I have set out with the aim of writing about my own experience from which I have gradually defined certain priorities and prejudices. These will not be everybody's idea of what is important but there would be little purpose in writing if every reader agreed with me and might, had they a mind to, have written the chapter themselves. That being so, I will spend a moment outlining the sort of work I have done so that the reader can put what is written into some perspective.

I have lived and worked with children with movement and/or developmental disability both before and since I became a physiotherapist 40 years ago and throughout this period have made cerebral palsy (CP) my primary interest. During that time I have examined around 2000 children with congenital or early acquired hemiplegia and watched many of them grow to adulthood. I have probably treated not more than a third of these children myself and then sometimes for not more than a year or so, but because I have worked in a tertiary referral centre and have also run an outreach service, there has been the opportunity to see the effects of my recommendations about aims and means of treatment as well as to observe the attitudes, treatments and outcomes of many other therapists, rather than just my own.

I think the three most lasting impressions of my experience are that, once beyond infancy, most of these children do very well with minimal but well-targeted intervention; that it is easier to tell from meeting the parents than from examining the child how much and what sort of treatment s/he has had; and lastly, the polarisation of opinions about what constitutes the correct physical management of these children.

At one extreme are those therapists who are constantly worried that they should be doing more, if only they knew what, to meet parental expectations and the apparent demands of this disorder. This attitude is partly induced by the teachings of the opposite extreme (which now includes special-needs teachers, conductors and others) who 'out-aim' the other therapists, confidently 'talking' such a good treatment outcome that they make all others appear to be unenterprising, out of date, ill-informed and defeatist. Too often in public debate, dissenting therapists, being perhaps less antagonistic, will lose out to this 'hard sell'. For it is easy to appear to treat CP well – it requires no more than the confidence to be dogmatic and a manner which captures the mood and aspirations of the audience: parents want to be told that there is an effective treatment for their child and inexperienced therapists need to hear that they can be instrumental in creating a more meaningful change. Outbidding other professionals may be easy, but it is somewhat more difficult to achieve the aims so confidently expressed; and it is uncertain if these aims are regularly, or ever, achieved because there have been few attempts to find out.

It has been argued that a child certainly will not achieve her/his best functional level if we set low targets. However, this hinges around what we mean by 'functional'. It is usually these same therapists we have been discussing who emphasise most strongly that the child is a person and not just a collection of disabilities. Yet childhood is finite – the time used for treatment cannot be replaced and there are so many other things to do which could be much more important for 'the person' than to be undergoing treatment. Before using up their childhood, be sure there is a good chance of worthwhile success.

Assessment for physical treatment/management

It is essential to know the things that will govern our treatment; and so we are looking for what limits function now and may be influenced by treatment or which may influence the aims or methods of treatment. This requires more than a physical examination as any treatment will have to take into account the intellect, personality and aptitudes of the child and the environment in which s/he is living. We also need to know the likely prognosis without treatment and some judgement must be made about the difference between that prognosis and one most likely after treatment. This can be done (imperfectly) only by experience and it will continue to need experience until we have the results of some complex research studies on the effects of treatment, which I suspect are many years away. We need to make some judgement about how much the child and family may 'lose' or 'gain' by devoting the time, making the effort, and enduring or enjoying the emotional strain of treatment. Treatment aims are best divided into the short- and long-term aims and the time commitment required to stand a chance of achieving them.

Lastly, some view on how the treatment might be delivered. For instance, will it be at the clinic or by visiting the child's home or school? How much can the parents take part? And so on. If the examination is of a child that someone else will be treating, then the circumstances of that therapist must be known: their experience, skills, aptitudes and back-up facilities.

Physical examination

TYPE OF MOTOR DISORDER

Most hemiplegia is described as 'spastic hemiplegia', indeed in some classifications it is the only description for a unilateral distribution of CP, but it hides a factor which has an influence on prognosis and so should affect the treatment. There appear to be three main ways in which hypertonia presents: velocity-dependent (spastic); non-velocity-dependent (rigid); and extrapyramidal ('dystonic') hypertonus. Many of the older children and a few from infancy have some component of rigidity in their hypertonus, but to simplify the description (and because it is irrelevant to what follows) this can be ignored. For a very few rigidity is the dominant component and then, in my experience, it can be very disabling and appears to be a marker for a more intractable lesion.

The real interest lies in the differences between the other two groups: spastic and what

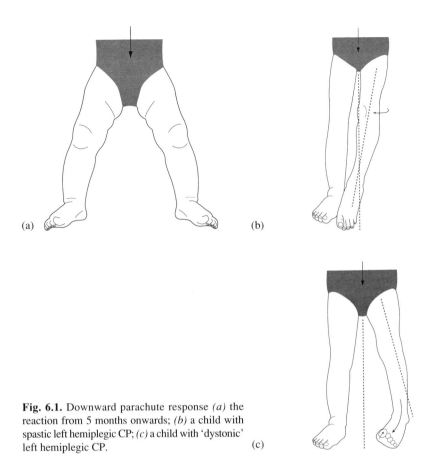

Fig. 6.1. Downward parachute response *(a)* the reaction from 5 months onwards; *(b)* a child with spastic left hemiplegic CP; *(c)* a child with 'dystonic' left hemiplegic CP.

I will call dystonic hypertonus, because in their pure forms they have different patterns of movement and postural reactions and so different prognoses.

Spastic hypertonus presents with brisk tendon jerks, ankle clonus, adduction of the hip as a response to a 'downward parachute' manoeuvre (Fig. 6.1a, b) and adduction of the hip on oblique suspension (Milani Comparetti and Gidoni 1967). These children prefer postures which tend to be away from the extreme in the hip, knee and elbow and lack an effective protective extension reaction in the arm (and less noticeably in the leg).

Children with dystonic hypertonus have normal or slightly depressed tendon jerks and effective protective extension reactions in arm and leg. The hip abducts and the ankle usually plantarflexes with foot inversion in response to oblique suspension and downward parachute reactions (Fig. 6.1c). The children tend to the extremes of inner- or outer-range postures and seem to find middle-range control a problem.

Just from reading the above, two differences may be immediately obvious to the reader. First, the sitting infant with a dystonic-type disorder will be able to achieve much more, as

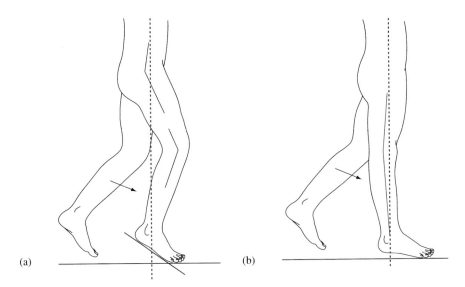

Fig. 6.2. Gait: stance phase. *(a)* right spastic hemiplegia and *(b)* right 'dystonic' hemiplegia.

her/his affected arm can act as a prop and save from falling, freeing the unaffected hand. The child with a spastic disorder, however, will spend much of her/his sitting time using the unaffected arm to retain stability. Secondly when walking, while both children have unilateral equinus (either postural or fixed), the child with a spastic disorder seldom makes an attempt to get the heel down (Fig. 6.2a) as the knee and hip 'prefer' to adapt by taking up semiflexed postures (the hip also adducts and internally rotates). Dystonic hypertonus induces a different gait: the child attempts to get his heel to the ground by hyperextension of the knee and retraction of the pelvis (Fig. 6.2b). Thus two distinct types of gait are produced, each with its own set of problems. A failure to appreciate this difference can lead to an ankle–foot orthosis (AFO) being made to the wrong prescription causing more harm than good. Each gait produces its own set of postural dynamics in the trunk and upper limb. Circumduction (swinging the straight leg through a lateral arc during swing phase to allow the toes to clear the ground – typical of later-acquired hemiplegia) is not a feature of congenital hemiplegia, apart from the small minority who have a predominately rigid hypertonus.

There is an additional characteristic to the natural history. Whenever a child develops a new skill those with dystonic hypertonia predominating exhibit much greater 'overflow' of posturing, which is gradually suppressed as the skill becomes more perfected. As a result these children usually appear at their worst at an early stage as each new skill is being learnt, but gradually improve. This is in marked contrast to those in whom spasticity predominates.

It is the dominant characteristic one is looking for, but a child may not fall into one group or the other and it is not unusual to find that, although both types of hypertonus are present in both the upper and lower limb, one may be dominant in the leg and the other in the arm.

DEFORMITY

Most babies born with hemiplegia do not begin life with any fixed deformity, but they do have a propensity to deformity wherever there is persistent postural imbalance due to hypertonus or skeletal asymmetry.

Fixed deformity

The term 'fixed' is used here to describe a loss of range of movement about a joint which cannot be overcome during clinical examination. There are two types: (1) limitation due to changes in the periarticular tissues and (2) lack of full extensibility of a muscle/tendon. In the latter, the joint range may vary with the position of a neighbouring joint if the muscle/tendon also acts upon (crosses) that joint.

Periarticular fixed deformity most often occurs at the ankle (equinus), wrist (flexion and ulnar deviation) and the radio-ulnar joints (pronation). There may also be fixed deformity of the foot and hand but these are intimately related to structural deformity (see below). Hallux valgus can become a major problem but it is secondary to hind foot valgus (usually equinovalgus) and the consequent change of forces at 'toe strike' or anterior rocker action. Fixed elbow flexion can occur but it seldom becomes the cause of functional limitation or comes to be more than mildly uncosmetic.

Structural deformity

'Structural' is used here to mean that the joint surfaces or bone shape have become altered by non-use or misuse. In the foot it is seen to be intimately related to periarticular changes in valgus or varus or as part of equinus deformity. In the hand small carpal changes occur related to the intrinsic and extrinsic forces usually associated with thumb adduction/opposition and wrist flexion/ulnar deviation. The other most common sites are the wrist, forearm, elbow, femur, tibia and spine. The upper-limb deformities have been mentioned already, but those in the lower limb require a little further discussion.

The hip joint of a child with hemiplegia seldom causes any problem itself, but its range of movement can be markedly affected by femoral neck anteversion. The term 'anteversion' seems to be the cause of much confusion and it is probably easier to understand its functional significance by calling it what it really is in a proximal-to-distal sense, femoral shaft internal rotation (or retroversion). This is because it is of little advantage to imagine an isolated femoral shaft having its upper end rotated so that the head moves anteriorly, when in real life (Fig. 6.3) it is the head which is fixed in the acetabulum and the distal portion which has to rotate in the opposite direction taking the shaft (and so the knee) into internal rotation. This bone deformity increases the range of internal rotation and reduces external rotation, but due to the geometry of the hip it has much greater effect when the hip is fully extended (and of course this is the more important position as it influences gait in a number of ways). Hip rotation should be tested with the child prone and his knee flexed to 90°, ensuring that the hip is extended. I have found that whereas children can stand comfortably with the hip near to its maximal external rotation, most naturally walk with it within about 10° either side of the middle range of rotation in extension. Thus if internal rotation were 80° and external only 20° the comfortable walking posture would be between 20° and 40° of internal rotation.

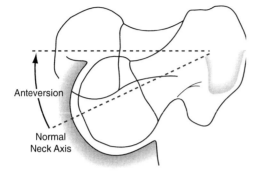

Anteversion

Normal
Neck Axis

Fig. 6.3. Diagramatic superior view of the upper end of the right femur and acetabulum. Anteversion of the neck is a (clockwise) rotation of the head and neck in relation to the femoral shaft; but since the femoral head remains within the acetabulum, this rotation affects the shaft and rotates the knee internally.

Any attempt to get the child to externally rotate more when walking will lead to rotation of the pelvis to the affected side (creating a false external rotation) or semiflexion of the hip (as even 10° of flexion greatly increases the range of external rotation). No amount of physical therapy can alter this situation.

Excessive torsion of the tibia, either internal or external, is not uncommon. It is measured most easily, and its significance best appreciated, by the thigh–foot angle as suggested by Staheli (1985). The child is examined prone with her/his knee flexed to 90° (Fig. 6.4) and the angle between the long axes of the foot and the thigh are estimated. It is important to have the foot in a corrected (normal plantigrade) position and not forced into valgus. The normal angle has the foot turned out by about 10°. Unlike the angle of tibial torsion, this angle changes little during (normal) childhood.

Some children develop external torsion as a compensatory mechanism to femoral neck anteversion, others do not and internal tibial torsion may increase the internal rotation of the foot position already caused by the femur. The foot angle is often the most noticeable feature when considering the gait of a child with hemiplegia and as efforts are usually made to achieve more symmetrical foot angles, a careful examination of the cause of in-toeing is essential: femoral neck anteversion, tibial torsion, forefoot adduction from an overactive tibialis posterior or a valgus foot are all causes, although sometimes there is no mechanical cause and it is a dynamic gait pattern, which may respond to treatment.

Hypoplasia

Hypoplasia of the affected side (hemihypoplasia) is also a structural deformity, but one which is intrinsic to the cerebral lesion rather than usage. It is a very common, but not inevitable, feature of hemiplegia. It can be (but seldom is) a major barrier to a socially acceptable static and dynamic posture as the arm, including the shoulder girdle, can be considerably smaller and more wasted than the opposite side; the trunk including the pelvis can be markedly asymmetric and the leg can be up to 4.5 cm shorter and wasted. It is essential that these structural aspects of the disorder are noted as they can set limits on what a physical treatment can achieve.

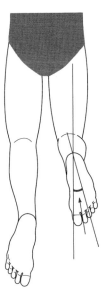

Fig. 6.4. Thigh/foot angle. Child prone, right knee flexed to 90°.

The only true shortening which needs to be measured is the leg. The other sites are hard to measure clinically and the leg is the one that can be, and may need to be, compensated by some form of shoe raise. However, it is not a simple matter of running a tape from the anterior superior iliac spine to the medial malleolus, as the bony landmarks (having different sizes and muscle forces acting on them) are seldom symmetrical right and left. By far the best method is to have the child stand with support if necessary and place graduated blocks under her/his foot. One is looking not for the anterior superior iliac spine to be at the same height, but for her/his overall posture to be at its most symmetrical. Yet the best gait is not always achieved with the theoretically correct static raise and, having established a base measurement, it is then a matter of trial.

One aspect of hypoplasia is that the true shortening in the lower limb is present very early and appears to alter little as the child grows after the age of about 2 years. This is important to the family who, hearing of 2 cm shortening at age 2 years may have a picture of their child as a young adult with 7 cm or more shortening and wearing a hugely raised boot. They need to be reassured about this, as it can be an unspoken worry. The shortening seldom changes by more than 1 cm throughout childhood and, of course, becomes an ever smaller proportion of limb length as the child grows.

Postural/dynamic deformity
These terms are used to mean almost the same thing: the deformity is one of postural 'choice' not of physical limitation (i.e. it is not 'fixed'). 'Postural' is used to imply a posture held preferentially when at rest and 'dynamic' for postural abnormalities which occur only with activity. Thus a child may stand with a postural equinus all the time or stand near-

plantigrade but adopt a dynamic equinus position only when walking or running or even when thinking of doing so. Persistent postural deformity may cause fixed deformity as the child grows.

The spine usually has a postural deformity convex to the unaffected side due to overactivity of the affected trunk side flexors. This may be exacerbated by a structural deformity of the trunk due to hemihypoplasia. However, when standing, the pelvis is often lower on the affected side which tends to produce an opposing curve. This pelvic posture is due to the true shortening of the leg (particularly if an AFO is used) or semiflexion of the hip and knee but, since equinus effectively lengthens the leg, it is apparent that almost any combination of spinal posture is possible. Severe structural scoliosis is rare.

'Catch positions'
These are closely related to dynamic postures. When examining the range of movement at a joint in the direction against the preferred posture it is best to move the limb segment slowly to avoid eliciting hypertonus; but having established the full range of movement, take the limb back to its original position and repeat the movement quickly. If there is any velocity-dependent hypertonus the limb segment will stop at a position well short of full range – the 'catch' position – and this is the position the child usually adopts during activity or excitement.

LOCOMOTOR DEVELOPMENT
The sequence of gross locomotor development is very likely to be different from the usual sequence, because the child will not find crawling an easy means of getting around and may adopt a position which is part side sitting (to the unaffected side) and part a shuffle (scoot). It matches their natural sitting posture and avoids weight bearing on the affected arm while allowing internal rotation of the affected hip, which is another preferred posture. Some children are natural shufflers and so would not want to crawl (or readily adopt a prone position) anyway. Sitting can also be affected by the type of hypertonus as this relates to the ability to prop and protect with the arm. Getting to standing is naturally done primarily by the unaffected leg and arm.Walking need not be delayed and can be early (7 months is the earliest I have seen), but most children walk at what is best described as late-normal and certainly can walk by the age of 2 years unless there is some additional problem or the child comes from a naturally late-walking family.

There is some evidence that left and right hemiplegia are not simply mirror images of each other and this is seen in gait. In a small survey of children in the age range 1 to 5 years with hemiplegia I found that gait asymmetry was characteristic of side (Scrutton 1976): the mean difference in foot placement angles (one measure of gait asymmetry) was 30° for the right and 8° for the left hemiplegia. In a series of 97 normally developing children this mean was 6° (Scrutton 1969). Indeed half the children with left hemiplegia had a difference of only 3° or less, whereas the figure for children with right hemiplegia was 29°, half of the normal series being equal to or less than 5°. However, in a group of 5- to 9-year-old children with hemiplegia, the mean for right hemiplegia was 6° and for left 8°; the mean for normally developing children being 2°. These figures suggest that gait development may be different and that high foot-angle asymmetry in children with right hemiplegia may be easier to correct or may even self-correct.

It is worth noting that in this same study of normal gait in young children that the length of the left step was frequently different from that on the right. Consistent step-length differences of 10% were present in 9% of the children. Perfect symmetry cannot be considered the norm, nor the treatment goal.

SENSORY DEFICITS
Sensory loss in the hand
Many children with hemiplegia have diminished sensory appreciation particularly apparent in the affected hand. All the usual sensory tests apply, but there is some discussion about how much it may be due to lack of experience (so-called 'virgin hand') and how much directly from the lesion. Clinical evidence leads me to consider that the predominant factor is a primary loss and that there is a frequent association between discriminatory sensory loss and hypoplasia (see chapters 5 and 9).

Vision
Apart from strabismus and hemianopia, visual difficulties are probably no more common in individuals with hemiplegia than in the general population. Although, since the child will have had a comprehensive developmental examination, any problem is more likely to be diagnosed. The hemianopia is usually to the hemiplegic side and may contribute to motor disability, particularly in infancy (see chapter 5).

Perceptual disorders
Anyone with CP is also at risk of disorders of central perception. A therapist needs to be aware of this possibility and a child who is functioning well below what might reasonably be expected from their motor disorder, general developmental level, vision and hearing should be referred back to the paediatrician.

EPILEPSY
Epilepsy is common in hemiplegia. Some drug regimen will adversely affect the child's overall performance and the frequency and type of fits needs to be known and borne in mind when treating (see chapter 10).

THE CHILD AND THE FAMILY
The purpose of the physical examination is to highlight what is in need of treatment ('need' here implying that it might respond to intervention, not a catalogue of all disabilities arising from the disorder); but it is also important to form some impression of how any intervention might be carried out. The child's personality and intellect are of obvious importance, as is the family's desire to cooperate and their relationship with the child. While most parents wish to do all they can to help in the treatment of their child, not all will wish to do so in the way the therapist thinks best and it is essential to find out how to work together in the best interests of the child. It is important to establish from the parents (and, of course, from

the child if s/he is old enough) what they expect and want from the treatment. Their immediate aims may be very different from the therapist's longer-term, and perhaps less direct, approach to a problem. Each of the following factors can affect the aims and mode of the treatment. If the child attends school, what is the likely cooperation and understanding of the staff in the classroom and for all other activities. For the older child, her/his interests and hobbies may be integrated within treatment.

One should also bear in mind how easy it is for the child to attend the clinic: is there good transport, do both parents work, can the child come alone, or are there other children to consider? One also wants to know if the child has been treated elsewhere. Was this a good experience? Were the previous aims and methods very different from your own? Is this going to be an advantage or predispose the family to perceive your approach as 'wrong'?

Treatment and management
Unlike most bilateral forms of CP, hemiplegia has a consistent and well-established natural history which allows certain clear statements to be made quite early on in the child's life. This is a great advantage to the family and in planning the treatment aims.

First, unless there is also a severe general developmental disorder or profound intractable epilepsy, the child will walk and do so by an age which will not affect other aspects of her/his general development. The affected leg will be used and the treatment will aim to maximise the efficiency and look of that use.

Second, in contrast the hand/arm can all too easily be ignored by her/him and take little (or a secondary) part in her/his life. The aim here then is primarily to ensure an early awareness of its existence and encourage its use, and secondarily to improve its efficiency and look.

Lastly, the spine may present problems, but these are unlikely to be major structural deformities and are more those of upsetting the child's postural static and dynamic symmetry. Except in the very few non-ambulant children, kyphoscoliosis is best considered as not being secondary to the hemiplegia and should be treated as a separate disorder.

THE 'WHOLE CHILD'
It became 'fashionable' about 40 years ago to discuss the treatment of CP as treatment of the whole child. For hemiplegia this meant that one did not treat the arm, the trunk or the leg, but the affected side of the body as a whole. It was not long before that came to mean both sides of the body being seen as part of a static and dynamic 'whole' (to the extent that some therapists even insist on bilateral AFOs); and shortly after that the child's developmental age and perceptual problems became part of the 'whole'. The current 'definition' includes the family/school/social environment. However, what seemed to be consistently ignored was the possibility that the treatment itself might be detrimental to the 'whole child and the family'.

It is my experience that many of the children are treated because they have hemiplegia, not because the treatment will be to their overall benefit. They have hemiplegia – we have treatment skills. Therefore, it would be wrong to withhold treatment. Any improvement to their physical function, however small, is seen to be to the child's advantage. This is nonsense, because it entirely misses out the detrimental effects which for some children can far outweigh the child's physical disability. Having a hemiplegia does not itself prevent a child from growing up to become an adult fully capable of taking part in society. In this sense it is quite unlike all but the mildest forms of bilateral CP. What prevents the child with hemiplegia from achieving this goal of adult social integration (which is, after all, the aim of the treatment) are three things: intellect, epilepsy and personality. The first two have little to do with physical treatment but the latter can be greatly affected by it. Many of these children become heartily sick of the continual emphasis on their deficiencies (of which they are all too aware) and being singled out as different from their peers by clinic visits and so on which do little to help them on their way towards a better self-image. They will willingly accept those things that obviously help them function better (provided these do not mark them out as being too different in some way), but have little time for the routine therapy which seems (and they are usually correct) to contribute little of importance to their way of life after the first few years.

When a mountaineer (George Leigh Mallory) was asked why he wanted to climb Mount Everest he is reported to have said, 'Because it is there'. It is all too easy for the treatment of hemiplegia to be based on that precept rather than asking if the overall effect on 'the whole child' is beneficial. The real outcome measure of treating children is the adults they become and childhood should be 'distorted' by treatment only where there is a good probability that the outcome will be worthwhile. The disadvantages can be too great for the therapist to continue to pursue small physical improvements which have no obvious long-term functional advantage.

What does this mean? It implies that the infant should get a massive treatment input and the ambulant child the correct orthotic and functionally beneficial equipment and training. It implies that those older children, who have appreciated that they have differ-ences which they wish to attempt to reduce or a skill they wish to acquire, should get a treatment planned specifically with the aim of achieving goals they have set themselves. Few children should be discharged totally from supervision; and being reviewed once each school holiday seems a sensible interval. It also prevents them from being seen to be different by missing school.

THE INFANT
Ideally the physiotherapy department will have close links with the well-baby clinic. However, asymmetry of any kind is easily seen even by an untrained observer and so a child with hemiplegia may be referred earlier for treatment than many of those with more severe bilateral disorders. Fortunately not all infantile functional asymmetry is permanent. Preferential head turning (Robson 1968) can cause marked asymmetry of function (neglect of the flexed 'occipital' upper limb and less movement in the 'jaw-side' lower limb), plagiocephaly and 'infantile scoliosis', all of which effectively resolve once the child can sit.

Children with something obviously wrong with them have anxious parents, who want to help them. For that reason alone early referral for treatment is desirable. Far from producing anxiety, it may allay it; and I remain convinced (in the absence of 'proper' evidence) that most of the children and nearly all of the parents benefit from early referral to a physiotherapist. Over and above this, if the baby is ever to be referred for treatment one of the first questions asked after the first treatment session is, 'Would it have been better if the child had been referred sooner?' and it is hard to answer, 'No' and still make one's efforts and advice seem worthwhile now.

Treatment during infancy has many advantages: there will not yet be any fixed deformity, movement habits are not well established, the baby needs to be handled and cared for and parents are prepared and expect to spend much time caring for their baby. So it is an ideal time to introduce therapeutic ways of handling the child which are advantageous to more symmetrical function, sensory experience and prevention of fixed deformity.

The aims can be summarised as encouraging (1) greater symmetry of posture and movement; (2) an awareness of the affected side; (3) prevention of fixed deformity; (4) support for the family.

Symmetry

Although the patterns of movement in hemiplegia may vary from child to child it does not take long to see which postures and movements predominate in a child. These are the postural habits we know the child will learn all too well and our aim is to give experience of the alternatives in the hope that these too will become part of the movement repertoire. Any means of stimulating alternative movement patterns may be used and at this stage of development and for these infants I have found the techniques of neurodevelopmental treatment (i.e. Bobath) by far the most applicable. Vojta (1984) implicitly and Katona (1989, and personal communication) directly state that their therapies, if started sufficiently early, can have dramatic effects in reducing (or possibly eliminating) the disorder of movement, but I have little experience of using their methods and don't consider myself competent to comment. It would be interesting to see if the prevalence of congenital hemiplegia in school-age children has been greatly reduced where these techniques are generally applied.

Awareness

Lack of sensory appreciation caused by inexperience is most likely in the upper limb and particularly in the hand, where it is most needed. It is easy for the baby to ignore the affected upper limb, but it is not easy to see how this might have a lasting effect, as (normal) babies with preferential head-turning, who may appreciate that they have a 'second' arm/hand only when they learn to sit at, let's say, 6 months appear to have no long-term effects (nor have I ever noticed any short-term effects after the first few days of using the previously neglected hand). It seems to me that it is much more likely that nearly all the cause of this lack of sensory awareness is central, but that does not mean that we should not be making the baby disproportionately aware of this side of their body and in particular their upper limb. The limb which gives me the least hope of success is the one which appears to have a lack of use disproportionate to a (mild) disorder of movement and the child's developmental age (see chapter 5).

Fixed deformity

Fixed deformity follows persistent postural deformity. Thus those with spastic hypertonus appear to be at greater risk of fixed deformity than those with dystonic hypertonus. The use of orthoses from the earliest age seems sensible: it does not preclude function, is of no social embarrassment to the child and is a visible sign to the parents that treatment is ongoing. It is also a more positive act to remove unnecessary orthoses than to introduce them later when it is apparent that fixed deformity is occurring. Parents should be taught full-range passive movements and make them a routine part of the baby's day. There are several reasons for this: it is part of teaching the parents about their child's difficulties – most parents will do something of this sort anyway and so should be taught to do it properly; it alerts the parents to any changes in movement range; the children appear to feel better for it; and it may even have some effect in terms of preventing deformity.

Hand splints need to be very well made if they are to be beneficial. A poorly made orthosis can impede function, fail to correct the posture sufficiently or at the correct joint (e.g. hyperextend the first metacarpophalangeal joint rather than prevent opposition of the first metacarpal).

The most likely lower-limb deformities are equinus and femoral neck anteversion. Persistent equinus should be corrected with an orthosis but whether one can so easily affect the anteversion (by controlling the baby's femoral posture) is less certain. There is little doubt that the persistent abduction/external rotation hip posture of floppy preterm babies causes marked retroversion, and so controlling the sleeping posture of a baby with hemiplegia may well be advisable; but I would not recommend any action which prevented active kicking when awake.

Support for the family

A family is usually more ready to accept a physiotherapist than many of those other professionals visiting their recently diagnosed baby. S/he can be seen to be doing something with a purpose and can also teach the family how to help their baby themselves. As with nearly all early childhood 'habilitation' it is better done in their home where the family are better placed to ask the questions which really worry them. A percipient therapist can be of great assistance in helping the family come to terms with this change in their life and, for children with uncomplicated hemiplegia, can be very positive in allaying most of the extreme family worries. Some of the more common issues which are discussed are: that their child will walk and walk effectively, perhaps at a normal age, but certainly not severely delayed; reassurance about leg length difference; and that there is nothing about the movement problems of hemiplegia which should prevent a near-normal and full life. The therapist should become a well-informed friend and allow them to express their feelings about their child, passing on information where appropriate (and with their permission) to the paediatrician. At the same time she needs to be aware that she is a guest in their house and is part of their lives not by right, but by virtue of her knowledge and experience.

THE PRESTANDING CHILD

The problem with the leg is not *whether* s/he will use it, but *how*. So it is important that

77

from the earliest age possible the child has experience of more normal use even if that is not what s/he will do when guidance is withdrawn. For example: getting to standing with assistance using the affected leg for the upward thrust, and bringing the other leg up beside it; supported one-leg standing on the affected leg, allowing and encouraging mobility in this position: up/down, rocking side to side and front to back all the time with the foot plantigrade; standing just on the unaffected leg, with the other flexed at the knee, abducted and rotated at the hip and then replaced on the floor for weight-bearing. I could go on, but the message is simple and does not need enlarging upon.

THE PRESCHOOL CHILD

This heading implies that we are dealing with a child who fills her/his day doing what is enjoyable and in doing so practises the movement synergies that come most easily and, more importantly, are the most effective. It is not a day which can be devoted to 'treatment' and indeed most of these children can 'smell an exercise' a mile away! This is the stage when treatment per se really has to be radically reduced if the child's (and indeed the parents') life is not to become one long battle. A battle which may do more harm than good; reinforcing the idea that part of the child does not work properly and that s/he is different in some respect from other children. One of the first impressions I had of adolescents with hemiplegia was that their greatest 'deformity' was 'a chip on the shoulder' and it is an attitude that many of them find hard to cast off in adulthood. It need not be so, and I suspect that much of what is done in the name of treatment (by well-meaning therapists, special-needs teachers and parents) is a contributory cause.

This does not mean that all treatment or physical supervision stops, but that there is a change of emphasis. Children who have had no treatment from infancy may well benefit from quite intensive therapy as they rapidly discover latent abilities; but this sort of progress does not continue. Those (as described here) who have been followed from early life are unlikely to gain more than they lose. It is at this point that therapy as such should change its emphasis from teaching how to move to showing the child how to function better; and this is particularly so for upper-limb use.

Lower-limb orthoses

So far as the child's gait and general posture is concerned it is essential that the affected leg has the best static and dynamic base possible: that is, the foot/ankle must be stable in an appropriate posture. When standing the feet are the points upon which the whole of the body's static posture is constructed; and when walking, the affected foot is the total dynamic base during stance phase, and during swing phase its posture can completely dominate movement in a search for consistent foot clearance. There are children with hemiplegia whose foot/ankle posture is adequate without any outside help and quite a large proportion, who need no more than that the ground reaction forces acting on the hindfoot are shifted medially or laterally with a heel float; but the majority cannot be expected to have cosmetic and efficient gait unless there is some orthotic control of their foot and (more particularly) ankle posture. Well-made modern AFOs allow this with minimal social impact and are readily accepted by most children simply because they work so well (a reminder to the therapist that a treatment which is really effective is seldom rejected by the child). However, there has to be a precise purpose in fitting any orthosis and while a 's/he needs an AFO' approach may be all right as an immediate clinical response, the prescription requires more clear definition before a cast of the lower leg is made; and that should include the type of footwear to be used with it. It is the orthosis which controls the foot posture, the shoe/boot is the interface which transmits the ground reaction to it and *together* they constitute the orthosis.

STARTING SCHOOL

One aim of all the preschool management should be that, by the time the child is moving out of the home and into school, no parent is feeling that their child is 'deprived' because the school has no physiotherapist. There will be many problems for their child facing up to the 'normal' world, but the family need to appreciate that separation from her/his peers with frequent clinic attendance or leaving class for treatment is not to the child's overall advantage. This process of weaning the parents off treatment (the child has no need for a weaning period!) has to start early and from almost the very start I try to build in the idea that treatment, however important now, will not be a permanent part of their child's life.

LATER TREATMENT

So our child, who happens to have hemiplegic CP, has moved on. S/he is now approaching puberty and has real interests and hobbies, aims which require, perhaps, really skilled movement ability. Now is the time to reintroduce treatment, but not as treatment. Whom does any child respect, listen to and emulate? Someone who is successful at the thing s/he really wants to be able to do: a first-rate violinist, snooker player, horse rider, footballer, dancer and so on. This kind of treatment is not a hospital-based procedure. Suggest to the parents that they find a class; enrol their child; explain to the instructor that not all may be possible and that this is not a sign of wilfulness or lack of intellect.

LEAVING SCHOOL AND BECOMING AN ADULT

In many countries the step from the care of the paediatric team into an adult world of health care can be a watershed experience. The paediatric physical therapist may also be part of, or work in close association with, the group of professionals who may now take on responsibility for the young person's physical management but often this is not so. It is essential that the needs of the child are carefully summarised in a written report and fully discussed with the young adult and her/his family. Those aspects of the young person's care which need monitoring, whom to see if and when a problem arises, and who is responsible for replacing any equipment which is broken or outgrown must be clearly written. The team or person who will have continuing responsibility should be contacted and an acknowledgement of that responsibility received.

Conclusion

Compared to most types of CP, infantile hemiplegia is a straightforward condition to treat and to manage. In the main it has an uncomplicated natural history and offers a reasonable prospect of a fulfilled adult life. Those children who have severe developmental delay, severe visual deficits or intractable epilepsy will have a very different life outcome; not due to their hemiplegia, but to other separate, although associated, pathologies. Infantile hemiplegia is not difficult to treat provided that the therapist (1) does not believe it is curable (and so understands that there is a limit to the effect of any treatment); (2) realises that this is a condition which, were the child to receive no treatment would, nevertheless, allow her/him to become an effectively functioning adult; and (3) appreciates that whatever else s/he does the child and their family must be helped to understand that we live most effectively by emphasising our assets and not by concentrating solely upon overcoming the deficits which we all possess.

Once these three precepts are fully appreciated, many of these children can be helped by well-targeted and closely monitored intervention which will benefit them throughout their lives.

REFERENCES

Katona, F .(1989) Clinical neurodevelopmental diagnosis and treatment. *In::* Zelazo, P.R., Barr, R.G. (Eds.). *Challenges to Developmental Paradigms: Implications for Theory, Assessment and Treatment,* Hillsdale, NJ: Lawrence Erlbaum Associates. p. 167–184.

Milani-Comparetti, A., Gidoni, E. A. (1967) Routine developmental examination in normal and retarded children. *Developmental Medicine and Child Neurology*, **9**, 631–638.

Robson, P. (1968) Persisting head turning in the early months: some effects in the early years. *Developmental Medicine and Child Neurology*, **10**, 82–92.

Scrutton, D. R. (1969) Footprint Sequences of Normal Children under Five Years Old. *Developmental Medicine and Child Neurology* , **11**, 44–53.

— (1976) The physical management of children with hemiplegia. *Physiotherapy* **62**, 285–293.

Staheli, L.T., Corbett, M., Wyss, C., King, H. (1985) Lower-Extremity Rotational Problems in Children. *Journal of Bone and Joint Surgery* , **67**A: 39–47.

Vojta, V. (1984) The basic elements of treatment according to Vojta. *In:* Scrutton, D. (Ed). *Management of the Motor Disorders of Children with Cerebral Palsy. Clinics in Developmental Medicine No 90.* London: Spastics International Medical Publications, p. 75–85.

7
GAIT ANALYSIS

Sylvia Õunpuu, Peter A DeLuca and Roy B Davis

The primary purpose of gait analysis in any clinical application is to provide objective documentation of gait and increase our understanding of the mechanisms of pathological gait. With this information, more informed decision making about treatment to improve gait function is possible. Gait analysis is also a very useful tool for the objective evaluation of treatment. Gait analysis does not, however, dictate specific treatment protocols. The final treatment decision is dependent on the philosophy of the treating physician.

Generally, gait analysis is appropriate for any person with a gait abnormality for which the mechanism and/or treatment is unclear. Unfortunately, the complexity of a gait problem may only be realized upon the examination of the gait-analysis data. At the time of writing, the primary routine use of gait analysis in the clinical setting is in surgical decision-making for the child with cerebral palsy (CP) (DeLuca 1991, Rose et al. 1991, Sutherland and Davids 1993). The large body of experience in the use of gait analysis in this patient population has led to major changes in surgical treatment (Gage et al. 1987, Perry 1987, Sutherland et al. 1990) – primarily the introduction of single-setting multilevel tendon lengthenings and transfers, and osteotomies. This approach has been possible through systematic study using gait analysis both before and after surgery.

Gait analysis, as defined in this chapter, consists of multiple components that provide a comprehensive body of information about how a patient walks. These components include the following:

(1) Clinical examination including assessment of passive joint range of motion, muscle strength, bony rotation, muscle tone and anthropometric measures

(2) Video recording of both sagittal (side) and anterior/posterior views with slow-motion and close-up capabilities

(3) Three-dimensional kinematics (segment and joint range of motion during gait) of the trunk, pelvis, hips, knees and ankles

(4) Three-dimensional force data and joint kinetics (joint moments and powers calculated from a combination of kinematics and force plate data collected simultaneously)

(5) Electromyography (muscle-activity patterns during gait)

(6) Temporal and stride parameters

(7) Energy consumption.

Each component as a stand-alone tool has specific limitations (Õunpuu et al. 1996). For example, temporal and stride parameters and energy consumption may provide an indication of function, that is, a very slow walking velocity and high energy cost would indicate a less than 'functional' gait. These measures, however, are outcome measures and provide no information about the actual gait problems and what should be addressed through treatment. Also, clinical examination measures, while important when severe contracture and bony rotational abnormalities are present, may not correlate well with gait abnormalities (DeLuca et al. 1998). Only with the integration of all the information provided by these measurement tools can the best understanding of the pathomechanics of a gait problem be reached. This will result in the most informed treatment decision.

There are many similar technologies available commercially for the collection of gait-analysis data (Davis and DeLuca 1996). Although a detailed description of these technologies is not within the context of this chapter, one point is worthy of discussion. Motion data can be collected and analysed with respect to two or three dimensions. A three-dimensional analysis, however, is necessary in order to accurately analyse most gait pathology as gait deviations (as discussed below) are not limited to the sagittal plane. Abnormal transverse plane rotations, which are very common in persons with hemiplegic as well as diplegic CP, can result in significant errors in sagittal-plane results if collected with a two-dimensional system (Davis and DeLuca 1996).

Gait analysis in hemiplegia
In hemiplegia, as with most neuromuscular disorders affecting motor control, deviations fall into several categories (Gage and Õunpuu 1989). There are typical primary gait deviations as a direct result of the pathology. There are secondary deviations as a direct result of the primary deviations and voluntary compensations on both the involved and non-involved sides. Finally, there are 'apparent' gait deviations possibly due to asymmetry which may confound the visual observation of gait. The purpose of gait analysis is to document the gait patterns and to help the clinician understand the causes of the gait abnormalities better by separating the primary from secondary deviations and compensations. Also, through the evaluation of pre- and posttreatment data, one can not only document the effectiveness of treatment, but can also better understand the contribution of primary versus secondary deviations.

There have been several attempts to use gait analysis to identify patterns of movement in people with CP (Winters et al. 1987, Kadaba et al. 1991, Sutherland and Davids 1993). The ultimate goal of pattern recognition is to associate a specific pattern with a specific set of treatments. Due to the complexity of motion (in three planes) and multiple levels of involvement (abnormalities at the pelvis, hip, knee and ankle/foot), categorizing each individual patient as one pattern is difficult. Identifying patterns at each joint and developing an understanding of the way the motion of one joint may effect the motion of others is a useful way to begin to understand the typical gait patterns in hemiplegic CP. Therefore, the following discussion of typical gait patterns in the patient with hemiplegia will examine gait abnormalities at several levels: (1) the individual joint in a specific plane of motion, (2) interactions across joints in an individual plane of motion, (3) joint interactions across planes of motion and (4) voluntary compensations. Examples will be given in each category.

A discussion of pathological gait is the most informative when using gait data presented in a plotted format. The examples of pathological gait for this section will be, in most cases, illustrated using the three-dimensional joint and segment kinematic plots. The kinematic plot provides a wealth of information about motion including the range (typically measured

Fig. 7.1. Sagittal-plane ankle motion showing excessive equinus in the swing phase and a double-bump ankle pattern in stance. The sagittal-plane ankle is the relative angle between the long axis of the shank and the plantar aspect of the foot as viewed by an observer looking along an axis perpendicular to the shank–foot plane.

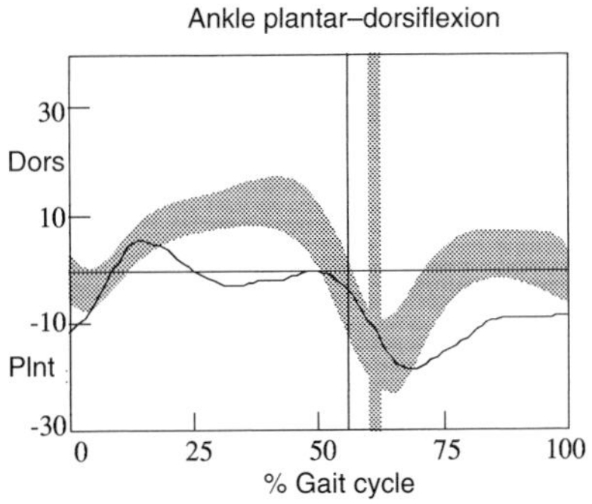

in degrees) and the timing of motion of a specific joint or segment over the gait cycle. The gait cycle is the period of time from initial contact of one foot to the following initial contact of the same foot. It is represented using a percentage of the gait cycle from 0% (initial contact) to 100% (subsequent initial contact). The plotting format for all the plots presented begins with the stance phase followed by the swing phase which are separated by toe-off indicated by the vertical line (Fig. 7.1). The normal expected pattern for each example is given by a gray band which represents a mean ±1 standard deviation. The angle definitions for each plot have been previously published (Õunpuu et al. 1991). However, a brief description for each joint and segment angle will be provided the first time a specific plot is introduced. The best way to understand a joint kinematic plot is to imagine a specific joint angle during gait being measured repeatedly and at short intervals and plotted on a graph over time. The individual points are then joined to form a curve which indicates the joint kinematic over the gait cycle.

Gait patterns in the child with hemiplegia
TYPICAL SAGITTAL PLANE DEVIATIONS
Excessive plantar flexion in swing (see Fig. 7.1)
Characteristics:
• foot drag at toe-off and initial swing due to clearance problems
• foot drop in mid to terminal swing
Possible causes:
• proximal weakness and instability resulting in clearance problems with associated foot drag
• heel-cord contracture
• inappropriate gastrocnemius–soleus activity in swing phase
• premature termination of anterior tibialis activity or anterior tibialis weakness
    A visual drop foot in swing does not necessarily indicate excessive equinus. Reduced knee extension in terminal swing and at initial contact can result in a down pointing foot (toe lower than heel) with a neutral ankle position. The sagittal plane motion of the ankle as identified with gait analysis can provide the most accurate confirmation as to whether the ankle is in a normal position in swing and at initial contact.

Excessive equinus in stance (Fig. 7.2)
Characteristics:
• initial toe contact
• absence or delayed heel contact in stance
• corresponding knee crouch or hyperextension
Possible causes:
• heel-cord contracture (may see absence of muscle activity)
• dynamic spasticity of the gastrocnemius–soleus (normal muscle length on clinical examination with plantarflexion in stance)
• rapid knee extension in mid-stance or hyperextension

Toe walking does not necessarily equate with excessive equinus. The ankle can achieve a normal degree of dorsiflexion in stance with only the toe contacting the ground due to greater-than-normal knee flexion. The sagittal plane motion of the ankle as identified with gait analysis can provide the most accurate confirmation as to whether the ankle is in a normal position in stance. Again, the position of the knee will have an effect on foot position.

Double-bump ankle pattern (see Fig. 7.1)
Characteristics (Rose et al. 1993):
• toe initial contact followed be immediate dorsiflexion
• this quick stretch on the spastic ankle plantarflexors is followed by premature plantarflexion (early heel rise)
• followed by a second dorsiflexion–plantarflexion movement in mid- to terminal stance
• plantarflexor moment (double bump in shape) over the entire stance phase (Õunpuu 1996)
• power absorption followed by generation absorption in mid-stance and power generation in terminal stance
Possible causes:
• dynamic spasticity of the gastrocnemius–soleus (normal or reduced muscle length on clinical examination)
• poor prepositioning of foot for initial contact due to less-than-normal knee extension which results in a flat foot on initial contact (ankle may be in a neutral position)

Excessive knee flexion at initial contact (Fig. 7.3)
Characteristics:
• greater-than-normal knee flexion at initial contact
Possible causes:
• hamstring spasticity and/or tightness (note: there is a minimal relation to the measurement of popliteal angle unless severe, i.e. greater than –80° of flexion) (Õunpuu et al. 1995)
• knee-flexion contracture
• poor ankle–foot control with preferred initial contact with flat foot (made possible by knee flexion at initial contact)
• combination of severe gastrocnemius tightness and use of an AFO that places the ankle in a neutral position with the remaining length of the gastrocnemius (double joint muscle) not sufficient to allow full knee extension

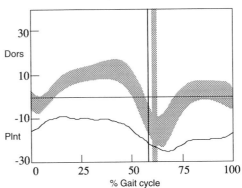

Ankle plantar–dorsiflexion

Fig. 7.2. Sagittal-plane ankle motion showing excessive plantarflexion in the stance and swing phase.

Excessive knee flexion (crouch) in stance (see Fig. 7.3)
Characteristics:
• greater-than-normal knee flexion in stance with associated increased knee extensor moment (Õunpuu 1996)
• less-than-normal knee range of motion in stance
Possible causes:
• hip-extensor weakness which reduces posterior rotation of the distal thigh segment
• ankle plantarflexor weakness allowing for excessive forward rotation of the shank segment
• severely tight hamstrings (greater than −80°)
• coactivity of rectus femoris and hamstrings (EMG for confirmation)
• knee-flexion contracture
• excessive heel-cord length allows for excessive forward rotation of the shank segment

    If transverse plane rotations are present, such as internal rotation of the hip, the knee may appear to be fully extended or less flexed visually or on the side view from the video recording. When this happens estimating the knee angle from a video recording will underestimate knee flexion. Sagittal plane motion of the knee as identified with three-dimensional gait analysis can provide the most accurate information as to knee position.

Knee hyperextension in stance (Fig. 7.4)
Characteristics:
• greater-than-normal knee flexion at initial contact
• rapid knee extension in loading response
• knee hyperextension in mid-stance with associated increased knee-flexor moment (Õunpuu 1996)
• net knee-flexor moment
• knee hyperextension on clinical examination
Possible causes:
• tight gastrocsoleus muscle which prevents forward motion of the tibia over the plantar grade foot (excessive plantar flexion knee-extension couple)

85

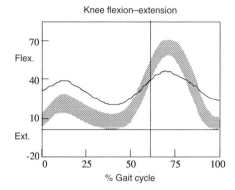

Fig. 7.3. Sagittal-plane knee motion with excessive flexion at initial contact and in stance. Angle definition for the sagittal-plane knee – relative angle between the long axis of the thigh and shank segments as viewed by an observer looking along the knee flexion–extension axis.

• forward trunk lean and anterior pelvic tilt, which brings the center of gravity forward, results in an increased external knee-extensor moment

Reduced and/or delayed peak knee flexion in swing (see Fig. 7.3)
Characteristics (Gage et al. 1987, Õunpuu et al. 1993)
• reduced peak knee flexion in swing
• delayed time to peak knee flexion in swing
• usually associated with clearance problems (foot drag in swing)
Possible causes: (most likely a combination of factors)
• rectus-femoris (knee-extensor) activity in mid swing (typically not vastus medialis or lateralis in persons with CP) (Õunpuu et al. 1997)
• ankle plantarflexor and hip-flexor weakness (in normal gait momentum into swing begins with the ankle plantarflexors and ends with the hip flexors)
• large knee-extensor moment with associated increased knee-extensor activity in terminal stance prevents normal knee flexion

Reduced hip range of motion (Fig. 7.5)
Characteristics:
• occurs on the involved side
• typically reduced flexion at initial contact and reduced extension in terminal stance
Possible causes:
• reduced disassociation between pelvis and femur
• hip-flexor spasticity which limits peak hip extension in terminal stance
• hip-flexor contracture which limits normal peak hip extension in terminal stance (a hip-flexor contracture in an ambulatory child with CP is rare, the measure may not be accurate if Thomas test is performed incorrectly) (DeLuca et al. 1998)
• hip-extensor weakness resulting in reduced hip extension in stance
• knee flexion contracture which reduces peak hip extension due to reduced posterior rotation of the thigh segment in terminal stance

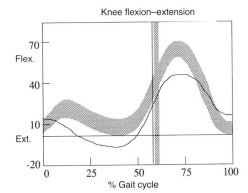

Fig. 7.4. Knee sagittal-plane kinematic with knee flexion at initial contact followed by rapid knee extension to hyperextension in mid-stance.

Due to difficulties in appreciating the position and movement of the pelvis in relation to the thigh during gait, hip motion is very difficult to estimate accurately on visual analysis. Motion of the hip (relation between the thigh and pelvic segments) as identified with three-dimensional gait analysis can provide the most accurate information about hip position during gait.

Single-bump pelvic-tilt pattern (Fig. 7.6)
Characteristics:
• gradual increase in anterior tilt in stance which reverses at about toe-off
• gradual decrease in anterior pelvic tilt from a peak just prior to toe-off to initial contact as the hip flexes during swing
• pelvic position at initial contact on the involved side is typically normal
Possible causes:
• reduced disassociation between pelvis and femur
• hip-flexor spasticity which results in increasing anterior pelvic tilt during hip extension when the hip flexors are lengthened (stretched)
• hip-flexor contracture which pulls the pelvis anterior when the hip is extending during stance
• rapid ankle plantar flexion in mid-stance which delays the forward motion of the tibia requiring anterior trunk lean and associated anterior pelvic tilt to continue forward progression

TYPICAL TRANSVERSE PLANE DEVIATIONS
The transverse plane is the most difficult plane of motion to interpret visually. The visual versus actual motion is often not consistent especially when there is asymmetry in pelvic motion in the transverse plane as typically seen in hemiplegia. Rotational abnormalities can occur through abnormal rotations of the hip, knee, and ankle joints as well as through bony torsion deformity of the femur and/or tibia. Finally, the pelvis may be held asymmetrically in gait, usually retracted (rotated externally) on the involved side in hemiplegia. Gait-analysis data allow documentation of all these potential sources of abnormal rotations. The typical transverse plane deviations seen in hemiplegia are summarized below and illustrated in Figure 7.7.

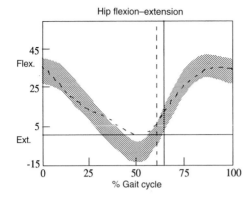

Hip flexion–extension

Fig. 7.5. Hip sagittal-plane kinematic with reduced overall range of motion in comparison to normal. Angle definition for the sagittal-plane hip – relative angle between the long axis of the thigh and perpendicular to the pelvic plane as viewed by an observer looking along a line connecting the anterior superior iliac spines (ASIS).

Excessive internal foot progression (In-toeing)
Characteristics:
• foot progression (as defined by the long axis of the foot) is internal to the direction of progression (i.e. the long axis of the walkway) in stance
Possible causes:
Primary
• overpull of the forefoot invertors (posterior tibialis)
• fixed forefoot adductus
Secondary
• internal rotation of the hip with normal alignment distal to the hip
• internal tibial torsion
• weight bearing on the equinus foot
    Excessive internal foot progression may also be present on the non-involved side as a result of internal rotation of the non-involved side hemipelvis.

Excessive internal hip rotation
Characteristics:
• on involved side
• femoral anteversion on clinical examination
• may visually not present as a problem as the knee may be pointing normally ('visually' simultaneous external rotation of the pelvis and internal rotation of the thigh segments can cancel each other out resulting in normal knee position in relation to direction of progression)
• gait analysis shows internal rotation of the hip throughout the gait cycle
• external rotation of the involved side pelvis
Possible causes:
Primary
• femoral anteversion (internal femoral torsion)
• dynamic internal hip rotation (muscle imbalance)
• overall lower-extremity muscle weakness

88

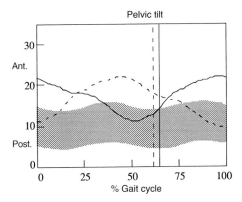

Fig. 7.6. Pelvic sagittal-plane motion for the involved side showing a single-bump pelvic-tilt pattern (dashed line) with increasing anterior pelvic tilt during stance and decreasing anterior pelvic tilt in swing. The pelvic motion for the other side (solid line) shows the reverse pattern. Angle definition for the sagittal-plane pelvis – inclination (typically forward) of the pelvic plane as viewed by an observer looking along a line connecting the ASISs.

External pelvic rotation

Characteristics:

• involved side pelvis

• external rotation throughout the gait cycle

Possible causes:

Primary

• reduced proximal control due to asymmetric tone with abnormalities on the ipsilateral side

• typically severe involvement of the ipsilateral upper extremity

Secondary

• compensation for femoral anteversion (as described above) to allow the involved side lower extremity to function in the direction of progression

• normal trunk tone with minimal-to-no upper-extremity involvement

CORONAL-PLANE DEVIATIONS

The patient with hemiplegia does not present with typical deviations in the coronal plane, although abnormalities in the coronal plane exist. Coronal-plane deviations of the pelvis are generally a function of the extent of leg-length difference. In those patients with a significant leg-length difference, with the involved side short, there is typically an obliquity with the involved-side pelvis down (depressed). This leads to relative abduction of the involved-side hip and adduction of the non-involved-side hip in stance. In some patients, where severe hip-abductor weakness is a problem, the opposite deviation occurs with the involved-side pelvis higher than normal during loading response (as the unsupported-side pelvis drops). There is simultaneous increased adduction of the involved-side hip in stance and abduction of the non-involved-side hip in initial swing to clear the stance-phase limb. In those patients with minimal involvement, the coronal-plane pelvis and hip show normal motion.

Joint-segment interactions

Motion of the segments and joints during gait are not mutually exclusive. This is why understanding gait deviations can become so complex. Reducing the causes of specific abnormal kinematic patterns to the muscles surrounding the joint alone is an oversimplification.

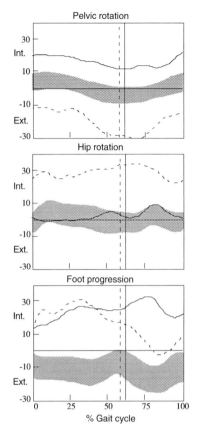

Fig. 7.7. Transverse-plane motion of the pelvis, hip, and foot progression for the involved (dashed line) and non-involved (solid line) sides. A typical pattern seen in hemiplegia is greater-than-normal external rotation of the involved-side pelvis, greater-than-normal internal rotation of the involved hip, and greater-than-normal internal foot progression, bilaterally. Internal foot progression of the non-involved side is a result of the secondary internal pelvic rotation on the same side. Angle definition for the transverse-plane pelvis – motion of the ASIS to ASIS line relative to a line perpendicular to the direction of progression as viewed by an observer whose sight-line is perpendicular to the pelvic plane; for the hip – the motion of the thigh (as defined by the knee flexion–extension axis) relative to the ASIS to ASIS line as viewed by an observer above the pelvic plane; and for the foot progression – the angle between the long axis of the foot (ankle center along to space between 2nd and 3rd metatarsals) and the direction of progression as seen from above.

Abnormalities at one joint due to muscle weakness, contracture, or control problems do not only affect the adjacent joint in the same plane of motion. For example, severe ankle plantar-flexor weakness which results in excessive ankle dorsiflexion in stance can also lead to excessive knee flexion in stance, but may also cause abnormalities at adjacent joints in another plane of motion. Some examples of these relations are discussed in the following section.

Increased sagittal-plane hip motion of the non-involved side (Fig. 7.8)
Characteristics:
• within-plane interaction
• greater-than-normal flexion in swing
• greater-than-normal extension in terminal stance
• greater-than-normal range of motion
Discussion:
This pattern is directly related to the single-bump pelvic-tilt pattern which is commonly seen in hemiplegia. To understand this mechanism, one must return to the angle definition

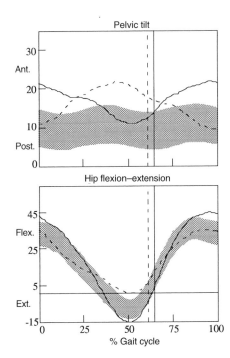

Fig. 7.8. Sagittal-plane motion of the pelvis and hip for the involved (dashed line) and non-involved (solid line) sides. The non-involved-side hip shows greater-than-normal range of motion due to the increased range of pelvic motion.

of hip motion which is the relative motion between the thigh and pelvis segments. When the hip is in flexion in swing on the non-involved side, the pelvis is in the most anteriorly tilted position resulting in increased hip flexion. When the hip is in extension in terminal stance on the non-involved side, the pelvis is in the most posteriorly tilted position resulting in increased hip extension. The net result is increased hip range of motion.

Excessive external hip rotation (see Fig. 7.7)
Characteristics:
• non-involved side
• within-plane interaction
• greater-than-normal external rotation of the hip throughout the gait cycle
Discussion:
This pattern is a compensation for the asymmetrical pelvic-rotation pattern with the involved side rotated externally (retracted) and the non-involved side rotated internally (protracted), which is commonly seen in hemiplegia. To understand this mechanism, one must return to the angle definition of hip motion which is the relative motion between the thigh and pelvis segments. When the non-involved side pelvis is rotated internally the ipsilateral hip must rotate externally in relation to the pelvis in order for the non-involved limb (foot) to point in the direction of progression.

91

Cross-plane interactions

Cross-plane interactions refer to deviations that occur in one plane as a result of a primary deformity in another plane. Three-dimensional joint kinematic data are useful in separating the primary deviation from the cross-plane interaction. The following example is a typical cross-plane interaction seen in the patient with hemiplegia who has a fixed asymmetry in pelvic motion in the transverse plane.

Asymmetrical hip adduction/abduction (Fig. 7.9)
Characteristics:
• seen on the involved and non-involved sides
• cross-plane interaction
• opposite and abnormal coronal-plane motion of both hips
• non-involved side – abduction at initial contact and adduction at toe-off
• involved side – adduction at initial contact and abduction at toe-off
• transverse-plane pelvic rotation is asymmetrical and consistent throughout the gait cycle
• seen when coronal-plane pelvic motion is symmetrical
Discussion:

This pattern is a secondary deviation seen in hip coronal-plane motion as a result of asymmetrical rotation of the pelvis in the transverse plane. Therefore, it is considered a cross-plane interaction. Again, to understand this mechanism, one must return to the angle definition of hip motion which is the relative motion between the thigh and pelvis segments. When the pelvis is rotated internally throughout the gait cycle, the ipsilateral hip must be abducted at initial contact to remain pointing in the direction of progression. Similarly, at toe-off the ipsilateral hip must be adducted to remain pointing in the direction of progression. On the opposite side, the reverse is true. When the pelvis is rotated externally throughout the gait cycle, the ipsilateral hip must be adducted at initial contact to remain pointing in the direction of progression. Similarly, at toe-off the ipsilateral hip must be abducted to remain pointing in the direction of progression. This asymmetrical hip motion will be eliminated with correction of transverse-plane pelvic asymmetry.

Voluntary compensations

Voluntary compensations usually occur on the non-involved side where the patient has the motor control to modify gait patterns and minimize the effects of the primary deviations. In hemiplegia, there are two examples of voluntary compensation on the non-involved side: vault and crouch. These problems do not occur simultaneously as the vault serves to functionally lengthen the non-involved side and the crouch serves to functionally shorten the non-involved side.

Vault
Characteristics:
• heel contact
• premature ankle plantarflexion in mid-stance (early heel rise)

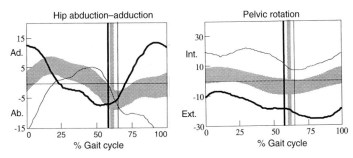

Fig. 7.9. *(a)* Coronal-plane compensatory hip motion for the involved (dark line) and non-involved (light line) side as a result of *(b)* transverse-plane asymmetry of the pelvis. The involved side shows greater-than-normal adduction and the non-involved side shows greater-than-normal abduction at initial contact with the opposite at toe-off. This asymmetry can be a result of a fixed asymmetrical rotation of the pelvis.

Purpose:
• to functionally lengthen the non-involved side to provide clearance of the involved swing limb which may be compromised by a drop foot and or limited/delayed peak knee flexion in swing

A vault during gait can look very similar to a spastic ankle pattern. The two very similar patterns can be differentiated by typically a combination of the following on the vault side:
• normal clinical examination
• heel-contact gait (dorsiflexor moment)
• normal ankle plantarflexion in terminal stance
• normal ankle power generation in terminal stance
• no drop foot in swing
• normal EMG in swing

Crouch (excessive knee flexion) at initial contact and stance
Characteristics:
• greater-than-normal knee flexion at initial contact and throughout stance
Purpose:
• to functionally shorten the non-involved limb length which can be significantly longer than the involved side
• minimizes the vertical excursion of the center of gravity and thus conserves energy
• can be decreased with AFO use on the involved side

Crouch on the non-involved side and pathological crouch can look very similar. A compensatory crouch can be differentiated by the following findings on the non-involved side:
• normal clinical examination
• normal knee motion in swing
• normal rectus-femoris EMG in swing
• elimination with lift or AFO (increases leg length) on the involved side

External pelvic rotation
Characteristics:
• external rotation of the involved side hemipelvis throughout the gait cycle (see Fig. 7.7)
• corresponding internal rotation of the non-involved side hemipelvis through out the gait cycle
• caused by greater-than-normal internal rotation of the involved-side hip (usually a result of increased femoral anteversion)
• compensatory external rotation of the non-involved-side hip
Purpose:
• to allow motion of the involved-side sagittal-plane knee within the plane of the direction of progression

During clinical decision-making, determining if asymmetry in pelvic rotation (with the involved side external) is a primary problem or secondary deviation may be difficult. If the patient presents with significant proximal involvement of the upper extremity and asymmetry in trunk tone, the pelvic asymmetry may not be a voluntary compensation. If they present with minimal trunk involvement, the pelvic asymmetry is most likely to be secondary to internal hip rotation.

Foot deformity in hemiplegia
In general, persons with hemiplegia are more prone to equinovarus rather than planovalgus foot deformities (DeLuca 1996). Also forefoot supination in terminal swing is a common finding. Assessment of these deformities should include a detailed clinical evaluation, radiographs, video analysis, and intramuscular EMG analysis (described below). Since the primary method of treatment of the equinovarus foot deformity includes multiple tendon transfers to restore muscle imbalance (Hoffer et al. 1985, Barnes and Herring 1991), electromyographic analysis is considered important to determine which muscle(s) are contributing to the deformity.

At the time of this writing, three-dimensional motion-analysis techniques are limited in their contribution to understanding the relative orientation of the hindfoot, midfoot, and forefoot. These difficulties are related to the small size of individual foot segments and the skin-movement artifact when dealing with relatively small movements. Therefore, information about the position of the foot during gait is limited to direct observations and the video recording. Close-up and slow-motion video of the patient walking towards and away from the camera can provide an excellent supplement to visual observation in the documentation of both the forefoot and hindfoot position during gait. Video recordings of multiple views of the foot and ankle during relaxed standing and during specific voluntary movements and the Coleman block test (Coleman 1983) can be a useful form of documentation.

Role of EMG in hemiplegia
Dynamic EMG is a common component of clinical gait analysis. Information about muscle-activation patterns during gait can not be achieved by any other means. The primary purpose of an EMG analysis is to provide information about when a muscle is active. Electromyography will also provide information about the content of a net joint moment, that is, whether there is simultaneous, antagonistic activity occurring. Unless normalized by a known force, EMG

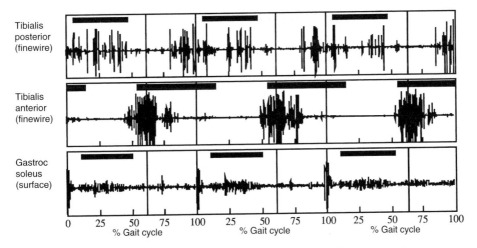

Tibialis
posterior
(finewire)

Tibialis
anterior
(finewire)

Gastroc
soleus
(surface)

| 0 | 25 | 50 | 75 | 100 | 25 | 50 | 75 | 100 | 25 | 50 | 75 | 100 |

% Gait cycle   % Gait cycle   % Gait cycle

Fig. 7.10. Typical EMG data (three gait cycles) for tibialis posterior, tibialis anterior, and gastrocsoleus in a patient with spastic hemiplegia. The posterior tibialis begins activity in the swing phase with variable activity in stance. The tibialis anterior is active at toe-off but shows premature cessation of activity in mid-swing with no activity in terminal swing. The gastrocsoleus is continuously active.

data do not provide information about the strength of a muscle contraction (Õunpuu and Winter 1989).

The use of fine-wire EMG for the examination of small surface muscles or deep muscles is common in hemiplegia for the evaluation of the equinovarus foot deformity (Perry and Hoffer 1977, Waters et al. 1982). In the treatment of equinovarus, a combination of muscle lengthenings and/or transfers is often considered. Electromyographic data can provide information about the cause of the foot deformity, for example, providing information about whether the posterior tibialis is active in the swing phase when it should be silent. Inappropriate activity of the posterior tibialis in the swing phase is a common finding in hemiplegia (Fig. 7.10).

Electromyographic analysis of the non-involved side in hemiplegia also can lead to some interesting findings. It is not uncommon to have 'abnormal' activity patterns of muscles in the non-involved side.

Clinical examination versus gait
The clinical examination is limited in determining the function of certain muscles and joints in a dynamic setting such as gait especially in disorders involving spasticity (Perry 1996). For example, in a series of 74 patients with spastic CP, the correlation between passive knee extension with the hip at 90° and knee extension at initial contact was $r = 0.32$ (DeLuca et al. 1998). The static clinical examination has limited ability to predict gait function for the following reasons:(1) the increased demands on the motor control system due to upright posture and balance requirements with resulting possible increase in tone and (2) the complex mechanics of movement during gait including the interactions across multiple joints.

Although the documentation of contracture and torsional abnormalities is important in clinical decision-making, the clinical examination as a stand-alone tool is limited.

Conclusions

The purpose of gait analysis is to provide objective documentation of gait and increase our understanding of mechanisms of pathological gait. Also, the comparison of pre- and postoperative gait-analysis data improves our ability to look critically at the effectiveness of a specific treatment protocol and allows a greater understanding of primary and secondary gait deviations. Although gait analysis allows for a more informed and perhaps more aggressive approach to surgical intervention, it does not dictate a specific treatment protocol. The final treatment decision is based on the treatment philosophies of the physician. Gait analysis in hemiplegia is a valuable tool which should be an integral part of decision-making for the treatment of gait abnormalities.

REFERENCES

Barnes, M., Herring, J. (1991) Combined split anterior tibial-tendon transfer and intramuscular lengthening of the posterior tibial tendon: Results in patients who have a varus deformity of the foot due to spastic cerebral palsy. *Journal of Bone Joint Surgery [Am]*, **73**, 734–738.

Coleman, S. (1983) Complex Foot Deformities in Children. Philadelphia: Lea and Febiger, p. 147–165.

Davis, R., DeLuca, P. (1996) Clinical Gait Analysis: Current Methods and Future Directions. *In:* Harris, G., Smith, P. (Eds.) *Human Motion Analysis: Current Applications and Future Directions* . Piscataway, NJ: IEEE Press, pp. 17–42.

DeLuca, P. (1996) The musculoskeletal management of children with cerebral palsy. *Pediatric Clinics of North America*, **43**, 1153–1150.

— Õunpuu, S., Davis, R., Walsh, J. (1998) Effect of hamstring and psoas lengthening on pelvic tilt in patients with spastic diplegic cerebral palsy. *Journal of Pediatric Orthopaedics*, **18**, 712–718.

DeLuca, P.A. (1991) Gait analysis in the treatment of the ambulatory child with cerebral palsy. Clinical Orthopaedics and Related Research, **264**, 5–75.

Gage, J.R., Õunpuu, S. (1989) Gait Analysis in Clinical Practice. *In: Seminars in Orthopaedic*s, pp. 72–87.

— Perry, J., Hicks, R.R., Koop, S., Werntz, J.R. (1987) Rectus femoris transfer to improve knee function of children with cerebral palsy. *Developmental Medicine and Child Neurology*, **29**, 159–166.

Hoffer, M., Barakat, G., Koffman, M. (1985) 10-year follow-up of split anterior tibial tendon transfer in cerebral palsied patients with spastic equinovarus deformity. *Journal of Pediatric Orthopaedics*, **5**, 432–434.

Kadaba, M.P., Ramakrishnan, H.K., Jacobs, D., Chambers, C., Scarborough, N., Goode, B. (1991) Gait pattern recognition in spastic diplegia. *Developmental Medicine and Child Neurology*, **33**(9), 28. (Abstract).

Õunpuu, S. (1996) Joint Kinetics: Interpretation and Clinical Decision-making for the Treatment of Gait Abnormalities in Children with Neuromuscular Disorders. *In:* Harris, G., Smith, P. (Eds.) *Human Motion Analysis: Current Applications and Future Directions* . Piscataway, NJ: IEEE Press, p. 268–302.

— Davis, R., DeLuca, P. (1996) Joint kinetics: methods, interpretation and treatment decision-making in children with cerebral palsy and myelomeningocele. *Gait and Posture*, **4**, 62–78.

— — Walsh, H., DeLuca, P. (1995) Sagittal plane pelvic motion: relationship to standing pelvic tilt and clinical measures. *Developmental Medicine and Child Neurology* , **37**(8), 25. (Abstract).

— DeLuca, P.A., Bell, K.J., Davis, R.B. (1997) Using surface electrodes for the evaluation of the rectus femoris, vastus medialis and vastus lateralis muscles in children with cerebral palsy. *Gait and Posture*, **5**(3), 211–216.

— Gage, J.R., Davis, R.B. (1991) Three-dimensional lower extremity joint kinetics in normal pediatric gait. Journal of Pediatric Orthopaedics, **11**, 341–349.

— Muik, E., Davis, R.B., Gage, J.R., DeLuca, P.A. (1993) Part I: the effect of the rectus femoris transfer location on knee motion in children with cerebral palsy. *Journal of Pediatric Orthopaedics*, **13**(3), 325–330.

— Winter, D.A. (1989) Bilateral electromyographical analysis of the lower limbs during walking in normal adults. *Electroencepholography and Clinical Neurology*, **72**, 429–438.

Perry, J. (1987) Distal rectus femoris transfer. *Developmental Medicine and Child Neurology*, **29**, 153–158.

— (1996) Function of the Hamstrings in Cerebral Palsy. In: Harris, G., Smith, P. (Eds.) *Human Motion Analysis: Current Applications and Future Directions* . Piscataway, NJ: IEEE Press, p. 299–307.

— Hoffer, M.M. (1977) Preoperative and postoperative dynamic electromyography as an aid in planning tendon transfers in children with cerebral palsy. *Journal of Bone and Joint Surgery [Am]*, **56**, 531–537.

Rose, S.A., DeLuca, P.A., Davis, R.B., Õunpuu, S., Gage, J.R. (1993) Kinematic and kinetic evaluation of the ankle after lengthening of the gastrocnemius fascia in children with cerebral palsy. *Journal of Paediatric Orthopaedics*, **13**, 727–732.

— Õunpuu, S., DeLuca, P.A. (1991) Strategies for the assessment of pediatric gait in the clinical setting. *Physical Therapy*, **71**(12), 961–980.

Sutherland, D.H., Santi, M., Abel, M.F. (1990) Treatment of stiff-knee gait in cerebral palsy: a comparison by gait analysis of distal rectus femoris transfer versus proximal rectus release. *Journal of Pediatric Orthopaedics*, **10**(4), 433–441.

— Davids, J.R. (1993) Common gait abnormalities of the knee in cerebral palsy. *Clinical Orthopaedics*, **288**, 139–147.

Waters, R., Frazier, J., Garland, D. (1982) Electromyographic gait analysis before and after operative treatment for hemiplegic equinus and equinovarus deformity. *Journal of Bone and Joint Surgery [Am]*, **64**, 284–288.

Winters, T.F., Gage, J.R., Hicks, R. (1987) Gait patterns in spastic hemiplegia in children and young adults. *Journal of Bone and Joint Surgery [Am]*, **69**(3), 437–441.

8
MANAGEMENT OPTIONS FOR GAIT ABNORMALITIES

Tom F Novacheck

Overview of the treatment philosophy

While the treatment of walking problems in congenital hemiplegia varies widely around the world, the following management scheme is used at the Gillette Children's Specialty Healthcare and Connecticut Children's Medical Center in the USA. The overall aim of treatment is to maximize independent mobility. Even though most individuals with hemiplegia walk independently, few do so normally. Some may expend more energy than normal (Bruce et al. 1994). In later years, pain or difficulty with footwear may be the focus of management. Surgical correction of foot deformity, patella alta, or hallux valgus may be warranted. In other cases, intervention is necessary to minimize the adverse effects of deformity or gait dysfunction on the individual's psychosocial function. The National Center for Medical Rehabilitation Research of the US National Institutes of Health model of disability provides a framework in which to understand the adverse effects of deformity on function.

Several salient points need to be made before discussing specific treatments. Physical therapy and orthoses are almost universally prescribed for children with muscle imbalance, spasticity, and the propensity to develop bone deformities and joint contractures. They are commonly prescribed at the time of diagnosis or shortly thereafter, usually in the second or third year of life. Muscles grow in length in response to the stretch applied to them by the growing bones to which they are attached. It has been shown that spastic muscles grow at a slower rate than normal (Ziv et al. 1984). In addition, children with delays in gross motor function do not put their joints in a position of maximum stretch as frequently as would typically occur during the course of play in normally developing children. Physical therapy to maintain or improve range of motion and orthotics to supply periods of stretch to specific musculotendinous units are generally used to counteract these potential ill effects. A knee immobilizer or an abduction orthosis can be used at rest to assist with positioning a joint to provide stretch to the hamstrings or hip adductors, respectively.

Orthoses may also be used dynamically during gait to provide stability to a joint, a stable standing platform during stance phase, improve ground clearance in swing phase, or assist with prepositioning of the foot in preparation for initial contact with the ground. The ankle–foot orthosis (AFO) is the type most commonly used. A variety of AFO styles are available. For individuals with cerebral palsy (CP), functional orthoses to assist with gait should seldom, if ever, cross the knee or hip joints. They tend to be too cumbersome, increase energy expenditure, and generally create more problems than they correct.

98

If a specific muscle group is particularly problematic in a young child (for example, developing contracture despite therapy and bracing), botulinum toxin injection may allow further maturation and delay surgical treatment until the child is older. It prevents the release of acetylcholine at the neuromuscular junction, and temporarily diminishes spasticity (O'Brien et al. 1995). Two types of botulinum A toxin are available – Botox™ and Dysport™. Due to dose limitations it can usually only be used to manage spasticity in isolated muscle groups such as gastrocnemius, adductors, or hamstrings (Cosgrove et al. 1994, Graham et al. 1995). It has several advantages over phenol or alcohol blocks. The injection of botulinum toxin is painless, produces no soft-tissue scarring, and diffusion throughout the muscle belly is rapid, eliminating the need for injection precisely at the neuromuscular junction. Its effects are temporary, lasting between 3 and 6 months.

Generally, it is best to delay surgical intervention until functional improvement reaches a plateau or the gait pattern has matured. This is usually at age 5 years or later. Recovery from surgery after the adolescent growth spurt is more difficult and healing is slower. Therefore, if surgery is to be done, the optimal age is between 5 and 12 years. As mentioned previously, the indication for surgery is usually to decrease the degree of functional limitation (the ability to get around in the community or to participate in everyday activities). The presence of pain, decreased endurance, difficulty navigating over uneven terrain or around obstacles, inability to progress to higher level activities like running, and the lack of normalcy of the gait pattern may also be reasons that families consider surgical intervention.

A detailed assessment must be completed to identify the abnormalities that adversely affect the child's function. This of course starts with the history, physical examination, and X-rays. The computerized information from the gait laboratory is an essential part of this assessment. Based on the evaluation, a comprehensive plan of treatment including surgery, postoperative physical therapy, and orthotic management is developed. An extensive post-operative physical-therapy program is essential to the success of surgery. If, for whatever reason, the postoperative physical-therapy program is unlikely to be followed, one should reconsider proceeding with the surgical plan.

Deciding who and when
To make decisions about the appropriate management of these gait abnormalities in the individual with hemiplegic CP, an analysis of the overall ambulatory dysfunction is needed. How does each of the gait deviations discussed by Õunpuu in the preceding chapter adversely affect the individual's overall level of function? To provide a framework, the attributes of normal gait (Gage 1991) must be considered. They are:
• stability in stance
• clearance in swing
• prepositioning of the foot for initial contact
• adequate step length
• conservation of energy

Are any or all of them lost or impaired? One must also consider what will happen with further growth.

TABLE 8.1
Common gait problems in hemiplegia

Primary	Secondary	Tertiary
Abnormal balance	Femoral antetorsion	Vaulting
Poor selective motor control	Tibial torsion	Circumduction
Weakness	Pes varus, cavus, adductus	Hip hike
Pelvic malrotation	Contractures – psoas, adductors, hamstrings, rectus femoris, gastrocnemius, soleus	
	Joint subluxations – hip, hallux valgus	

Abnormal gait can be caused by primary anomalies, secondary deformities, and tertiary coping responses or compensations (Gage 1991). These are listed in Table 8.1. Some of the prerequisites for normal gait can be lost in hemiplegia due to the primary and secondary abnormalities. The patient may use tertiary compensations in an effort to maintain maximum function and energy efficiency. The clinician must be able to distinguish between these since treating the primary and secondary problems will eliminate the need for the tertiary compensation. It will, therefore, disappear. Inappropriately treating the tertiary compensation would worsen the gait pattern. For example, a drop foot on the involved side in swing will lead to inadequate swing-phase clearance (one of the attributes of normal gait). The patient may compensate by vaulting on the contralateral side. If the surgeon fails to recognize this as an appropriate coping response and surgery is done to lengthen the heel cord on the contralateral side, the coping mechanism is ablated, and the patient's function will worsen. On the other hand, if the drop foot is appropriately treated with an AFO or tendon transfer, the compensatory vault will disappear as it is no longer necessary. The gait analysis laboratory is the tool that is invaluable in accurately identifying these issues.

Unfortunately, clinicians do not currently have the ability to completely correct or even significantly alter many of the primary problems. Many children (and their families) or young adults wonder whether something can be done to improve their ambulatory function and/or normalize their gait pattern. By dissecting the gait deviations in the gait analysis laboratory, one can begin to have the knowledge necessary to counsel the patient and the family as to what, if anything, can or should be done. The patient and family must be counseled as to what portions of the pathology can be treated and which ones will remain despite intervention. We have found it useful to review the list of problems in Table 8.2 with the patient and family prior to proceeding with treatment. The reader will recognize these as another way to subdivide the primary, secondary, and tertiary problems listed earlier. By discussing the patient's specific problems in each of these areas, expectations will hopefully be more realistic leading to both better decision-making and a greater degree of satisfaction with the outcome. For instance, surgery cannot improve selective motor control. That problem will remain after surgical treatment. The impact that this residual problem will have on the final outcome must be appreciated prior to treatment. The surgeon must also realize that a

TABLE 8.2
Gait problems in cerebral palsy (a helpful list for patient education)

Categories	Examples
Abnormal tone	Spasticity – manual control center
	Dystonia – automatic control center
Muscle contractures and/or abnormal bone growth	Foot deformities
	Hip dislocation or subluxation
	Torsional deformities of long bones
Problems with balance	Central from the brain
	From an abnormal base of support
Loss of selective motor control	-
Substitution of patterned movements from other brain centers to replace lost function	Pelvic malrotation
	Some cases of crouch

patient whose gait is characterized by an abnormal patterned movement will improve less with surgical treatment than someone who has a higher degree of selective motor control. This can be particularly true of patients with severe hemiplegia who have poor selective motor control and whose gait pattern may not change significantly following surgery.

The multiple lower-extremity procedure (MLEP)

If surgery is planned, the correctable biomechanical abnormalities are addressed by performing appropriate surgical procedures under one anaesthetic. Often multiple abnormalities are corrected. At our hospital, the Gillette Children's Specialty Healthcare, St. Paul, MN, USA, this is referred to as an MLEP (multiple lower-extremity procedure). Between three and seven procedures is typical of the number of procedures to be carried out. Postoperative immobilization is minimized as much as possible allowing the patient to rapidly regain functional independence, minimizing weakness, and avoiding decreased range of motion. Usually cast immobilization is necessary for 3 to 8 weeks depending on the patient's age and on the procedures performed. Weightbearing generally begins 3 to 4 weeks postoperatively in orthotics or casts. Molds for customized orthotics are made at the time of surgery or at the first postoperative visit. The orthotic is fitted at the completion of cast immobilization.

Physical therapy to maximize muscle strength and joint range of motion is an integral part of the rehabilitation program. Initial therapy is 2 to 3 times per week and is ultimately tapered to once per week depending upon progress. With time, maximizing functional skills becomes the focus of the rehabilitation program.

Postoperative management to maturity

Postoperative gait analysis is performed 9 to 12 months after surgery provided rehabilitation is complete. This allows an assessment of the outcome of treatment, provides guidance for

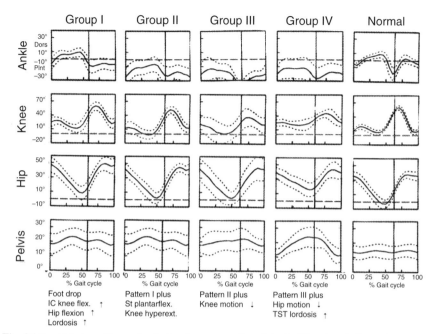

Fig. 8.1 Sagittal plane kinematics in the four types of hemiplegia. The plots indicate the mean (solid line) and the standard deviations (dotted line) of sagittal-plane joint motions for each group and for a group of individuals without hemiplegia (Reproduced with permission of Winters et al. 1987).

the continued use of orthotics during gait, and occasionally indicates the need for small additional operative procedures to optimize function. If hardware was implanted at the time of the MLEP, any additional surgery can be performed in conjunction with hardware removal.

To prevent recurrence of deformity or contracture during the remaining years of growth, a stretching program with or without night splinting is continued. Occasionally botulinum toxin is used to maintain appropriate muscle length especially during periods of rapid skeletal growth. If this program of stretching, splinting, improved functional mobility, and botulinum toxin injection is successful, the potential for repeat surgery is minimized

Recognizing gait patterns in hemiplegia

Penny has described a proximal-to-distal pattern of recovery of locomotor function following injury to the developing brain (Perry et al. 1978). If recovery is incomplete, a fixed limb synergy pattern persists distally. Based on this concept, Winters and colleagues (Winters et al. 1987) described four patterns of involvement based on sagittal-plane kinematic abnormalities (Fig. 8.1).

More recently, our laboratory has confirmed distinguishing characteristic sagittal-plane kinetic data (Bruce et al. 1994). In addition, oxygen cost and consumption data show a trend of increasing usage with increasing severity according to subtype confirming greater inefficiency with greater involvement. The children with less severe forms have distal abnormalities (ankle). As severity increases, abnormalities are seen at more proximal joints (i.e. knee [Type III] and hip [Type IV]). More severe levels of involvement share all of the distal abnormal features of the less severe levels. When considering surgery, corrections must incorporate all of the corrections of the lower levels. In this way they are additive as the level of involvement ascends from the ankle to the knee to the hip.

This classification scheme is based on abnormalities in sagittal-plane kinematics. It is important to recognize that these patients often also have secondary long-bone torsional deformities related to delays in development and abnormal biomechanical stresses (see Table 8.1). These deformities can be present on either the hemiplegic or the less involved side. Occasionally these deformities may make it difficult to determine if there is any neurological abnormality on the opposite non-involved side. The gait analysis laboratory is particularly useful for shedding light on these issues. As in other types of CP, correction of the long-bone torsions (femoral or tibial derotational osteotomies) as well as foot deformities may be an essential component of the management plan to improve mobility.

Surgical management will be addressed in two sections. Sagittal-plane problems will be discussed in the next section. Bone and foot deformities are identified primarily in the transverse plane and will be presented in the second section.

Treatment based on subtype (sagittal-plane considerations)
TYPE I
The principal problem with Type I involvement is a drop foot in swing phase. There is relative overactivity of the gastrocnemius–soleus compared to the anterior tibial musculature leading to swing-phase dysfunction. These patients have problems with poor swing-phase clearance and poor prepositioning for initial contact (IC). Initial contact is foot flat or on the toe. Therefore, first rocker is absent, and second rocker begins at IC. There is no limitation of ankle dorsiflexion in stance (the crucial distinction between this subtype and Type II). This pattern represents an individual who has 'regained voluntary control of the hip and knee, but not the ankle, which is still tied to the extensor locomotor pattern' (Gage 1991, p. 135).

Treatment is directed at restoration of clearance in swing phase and prepositioning of the foot for IC. This can be done most easily using a posterior leaf-spring ankle–foot orthosis since the gastrocsoleus can achieve a normal length.

The imbalance between the ankle plantarflexors and dorsiflexors can sometimes also be improved by transferring the flexor digitorum longus to the dorsum of the foot through the interosseus membrane. This procedure was originally described by Hiroshima and coworkers (Hiroshima et al. 1988) and included a transfer of the flexor hallucis longus as well. We have preferred instead to transfer the flexor digitorum longus alone. Results tend to be somewhat unpredictable. Some gain voluntary motor control of the transferred tendon, some have improved swing-phase dorsiflexion without active control, and some show little apparent improvement.

TYPE II
Abnormal stance phase function of the ankle plantarflexors distinguishes Type II from Type I. Ankle plantarflexion is excessive throughout the gait cycle. A static or dynamic contracture

of the triceps surae and tibialis posterior is present. This leads to equinovarus deformity. In addition to the Type I problems, poor clearance in swing and inappropriate prepositioning for initial contact, instability in stance is present. Weightbearing forces are distributed abnormally across the plantar aspect of the foot being concentrated along its lateral border.

In young children, an AFO can be used. Botulinum toxin injection can help maintain braceability. In older children in whom more conservative measures are no longer effective, lengthening of the gastrocnemius muscle corrects equinus positioning. Occasionally, the soleus may also be contracted and a lengthening of its fascia may also be necessary. We prefer not to perform lengthenings of the Achilles tendon since it probably overlengthens the soleus muscle and underlengthens the two joint gastrocnemius muscle. Potential force production by the soleus is extremely sensitive to lengthening. A 1 cm lengthening of the muscle causes a 50% decrease in its force generating capability (Delp and Zajac 1992). Appropriate individual lengthenings of each muscle/tendon unit can be performed through the same incision in the midcalf. Gastrocnemius recession (Strayer 1950, Baker 1956) has been shown to improve ankle modulation while preserving the power-generating capabilities of the muscles about the ankle (Rose et al. 1993). If contracture of the soleus remains after gastrocnemius recession, the fascia and central raphe of the soleus, which lie directly beneath the lengthened gastrocnemius fascia, can be lengthened. Just as in Type I, an Hiroshima transfer may help with ankle dorsiflexion in swing.

TYPE III

Abnormal neurological function persists that adversely affects the musculature about the knee, the hamstrings and rectus femoris. Hamstring spasticity or contracture can produce functional leg-length discrepancy by causing unilateral stance-phase flexion. Coping responses are then needed to preserve gait efficiency. Step length is shortened as the knee does not extend fully in swing. It is at this level of hemiplegic involvement that all five prerequisites of normal gait are lost.

Rectus femoris spasticity or contracture causes a stiff knee in swing and exacerbates swing-phase clearance problems. The overall range of knee motion is restricted due to cospasticity of these antagonist muscles.

Hamstrings

Treatment may include stretching casting in the very young child if the standard program of stretching is unable to maintain adequate length of the musculotendinous unit. The stretching program may be supplemented by botulinum toxin injection. Fractional medial hamstring lengthening is necessary in the older child to treat progressive musculotendinous contracture. Lateral lengthening is generally only required in more mature individuals with fixed knee-flexion contracture in which case postoperative dropout casting is often necessary to stretch posterior capsular tightness. In severe cases, posterior knee capsular release or distal femoral extension osteotomy may be required.

Semitendinosis transfer to the distal femur may be useful in preserving the important role of the hamstrings as hip extensors when medial and lateral hamstring lengthening is necessary. This has not been proven and the role of this procedure is debatable. As originally described by Eggers (1952), multiple hamstring tendons were divided from their insertions on the proximal tibia and transferred to the femoral condyles. This procedure proved to be excessive. Recently, transfer of the semitendinosus alone has been advocated. Experience with this procedure at Newington Children's Hospital (Newington, CT; now part of Connecticut Children's Medical Center) has shown that the semitendinosus transfer may excessively shorten the step length by tethering the femur and decreasing hip flexion (unpublished data). If the transfer is performed with excessive tension on the musculotendinous unit, and the length of the tendon is excessively shortened, its spring-like properties are lost. Preserving tendon length and avoiding excessive tension may address this issue and increase the utility of this procedure.

Generally hamstring overactivity or contracture has been considered to be the cause of crouch gait. Recent research has directed attention away from hamstring shortness as the etiology for crouch gait in many patients with spastic diplegic CP. Hoffinger and colleagues (Hoffinger et al. 1993) found that in the majority of their patients walking in crouch the hamstrings were longer than normal during gait! This work suggests that hip-flexion deformity and anterior pelvic tilt displace the hamstring origin proximally causing a secondary knee-flexion deformity. This phenomenon has been dubbed 'hamstring shift'. If this is true, then more attention should be paid to correcting hip-flexion deformity and anterior pelvic tilt than to hamstring tendon lengthening.

Rectus femoris
Distal rectus femoris transfer is the most effective treatment for this problem (Gage et al. 1987). It can be transferred to the sartorius or the gracilis with equivalent results (Õunpuu et al. 1993a, Chung, et al. 1997) This author prefers the suture repair to the tendinous structure of the gracilis rather than to the muscle belly of the sartorius. The rectus femoris normally acts as a hip flexor/knee extensor. Following the transfer it is changed to a hip flexor/knee flexor and inappropriate activity of the rectus during swing phase will now augment rather than hinder knee flexion. Some authors have advocated rectus femoris release rather than transfer. Sutherland and coworkers (Sutherland et al. 1990) have shown greater improvement with transfer. Release should not be done if knee range of motion is less than 80% of the normal range (Õunpuu et al. 1993b). It should also be noted that hamstring lengthening without rectus femoris transfer results in skewing of the knee flexion–extension curve towards extension (Gage et al. 1987).

TYPE IV
The hip flexors and adductors function abnormally with this degree of persistent neurologic dysfunction. All of the problems below are exacerbated by the dysfunction about the hip. Surgical intervention may include psoas lengthening. For treatment of the psoas, we prefer intramuscular lengthening of the tendon at the pelvic brim. The psoas is an essential power generator in normal walking. This procedure effectively lengthens the contracted psoas tendon while preserving its role as a hip flexor to propel the leg into swing (Novacheck et al. 1996). Release of the tendon from the lesser trochanter ablates this capability (Bleck and Holstein 1963).

The adductors have an important stabilizing function in walking and like the psoas

105

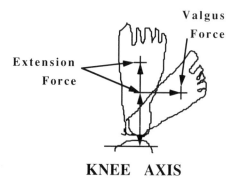

KNEE AXIS

Fig. 8.2 Lever Arm disease (Novacheck 1996). If an external foot-progression angle exists because of an external tibial torsion, the plantarflexion moment produced by the gastrocsoleus is diminished because the length of the moment arm is diminished in the sagittal plane.

may be useful for limb advancement. This is especially true on the hemiplegic side because the pelvis is generally rotated externally (retracted). In this position, contraction of the adductors advances the limb in the line of progression. Ablative surgery is to be avoided as it can be disabling. Surgical intervention generally is limited to division of the adductor longus at its origin and distal lengthening of the intramuscular gracilis tendon. Obturator neurectomy should never be done in an ambulatory child. Postoperative positioning with an abductor pillow and a physical therapy stretching program are important.

Management of bone and foot deformities
(Transverse-plane considerations)
Transverse-plane abnormalities of the lower extremities in all forms of CP are quite common and can in fact affect the uninvolved side in hemiplegia. Common deformities in hemiplegia include excessive femoral antetorsion, external tibial torsion, and midfoot adductus. Unfortunately, these deformities are often not adequately recognized, and their impact on gait dysfunction not fully appreciated. These types of bone deformities can lead both to problems with instability as well as poor clearance. In addition, the importance of bone deformity lies in the creation of lever arm disease (Novacheck 1996). According to this concept, a muscle's ability to create a moment about a joint is diminished if the bone is deformed (Fig. 8.2).

EXCESSIVE FEMORAL ANTETORSION
The femoral neck normally lies in the coronal plane maximizing the moment-generating capability of the hip abductors Femoral antetorsion alters the orientation of the femur leading to hip abductor insufficiency (Novacheck 1996).
    Correction is indicated if external rotation is insufficient to maintain a normal foot-progression angle, the hip is subluxated, or the antetorsion is greater than 40 to 45°.

106

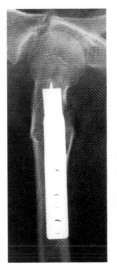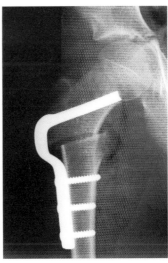

Fig. 8.3 Intertrochanteric femoral
osteotomy.

Correction is generally performed proximally at the intertrochanteric level, but supracondylar correction is also possible (Novacheck 1996). For the intertrochanteric correction, AO blade plate fixation is used (Root and Diegal 1980) (Fig. 8.3).

EXTERNAL TIBIAL TORSION

External tibial torsion develops later than femoral antetorsion. It is a result of an abnormal external rotation torque on the distal tibial physis. This is often due to the combination of poor clearance with resultant toe dragging and femoral antetorsion. The consequence is an external foot-progression angle. Figure 8.4 illustrates the kinematic abnormalities seen in combined femoral antetorsion and external tibial torsion.

Tibial derotational osteotomy corrects the deformity (Novacheck 1996). Representative radiographs are seen in Figure 8.5. To prevent recurrence one must correct the etiologic mechanism by performing a femoral derotation, hamstring lengthening, and rectus transfer if indicated.

Correction is indicated if the malrotation causes instability in stance or if the plantarflexor moment is inadequate to prevent crouch gait. If the foot is malrotated, crouch can result and may be progressive as the soleus can no longer generate an adequate plantarflexor moment to control the forward movement of the tibia over the stationary foot. The plantarflexion moment produced by the gastrocsoleus may be diminished because the length of the moment arm is diminished in the sagittal plane (see Fig. 8.2). Correction of this bone deformity improves plantarflexion moment generation.

COMMON FOOT DEFORMITIES IN HEMIPLEGIA

Metatarsus adductus can contribute to transverse plane malalignment during gait. It is fairly common in hemiplegia, is apparent on physical examination, and is confirmed with

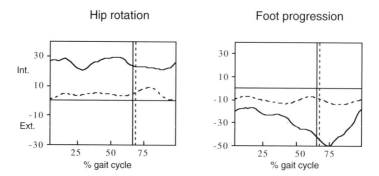

Fig. 8.4 Transverse plane kinematic abnormalities due to combined excessive femoral anteversion and external tibial torsion.

standing radiographs. Supple deformities at younger ages may be controlled with an AFO. Generally this deformity is rigid by the time a patient comes to surgical treatment, and corrective osteotomy is required. One option is multiple metatarsal osteotomies. Lateral column shortening (closing-wedge osteotomy of the cuboid) alone or in conjunction with medial column lengthening (opening-wedge osteotomy of the first cuneiform – the resected portion of the cuboid works well) is also a good option (Kling et al. 1991).

Some patients actually have a 'triple twist' deformity in their lower extremities – excessive femoral antetorsion, external tibial torsion, and metatarsus adductus. Individuals with this degree of complexity challenge the surgeon's decision-making ability!

While pes planovalgus deformity with midfoot break is common in diplegia and quadriplegia, the more frequent hindfoot deformity in hemiplegia is pes varus. This deformity can cause instability in stance due to excessive lateral weight bearing. Overactivity of the posterior tibialis is generally the cause. Correction can be obtained by soft-tissue balancing alone in the younger patient, potentially including posterior tibialis intramuscular lengthening (Frost 1971) and plantar fascia release. Split posterior tibial tendon transfer is another option (Green 1992). In the older patient with a fixed deformity, Dwyer lateral closing-wedge osteotomy of the calcaneus can be combined with soft-tissue rebalancing procedures (Dwyer 1959). Triple arthrodesis should be reserved for the most severe deformities in those with a more limited level of function. Transfers of the posterior tibialis through the interosseus membrane to the dorsum of the foot can lead to calcaneus deformity in the long term and should not be done.

Pes cavus may occur in isolation, but is more commonly seen in conjunction with other foot deformities such as varus (therefore, a cavovarus foot) or adductus (cavoadductus). Plantar fascia stripping is useful to correct this deformity. With severe, rigid deformities a dorsal closing-wedge osteotomy of the midfoot may be necessary (Tachdjian 1990).

LEG-LENGTH DISCREPANCY (LLD)
While LLD is common, it is usually 1 centimeter or less. The hemiplegic side is always

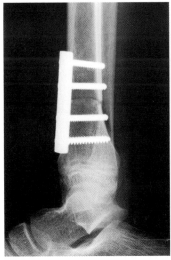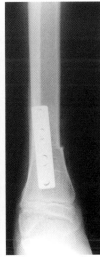

Fig. 8.5 Supramalleolar tibial derotational osteotomy.

the shorter leg. This degree of discrepancy is well tolerated and in fact may be beneficial in diminishing swing-phase clearance problems. Occasionally, the difference can be larger warranting treatment. One must always be aware of the compounding effect of a knee-flexion contracture on the measurement of leg length. A supine scanogram cannot account for this deformity; therefore, a CT scan may be necessary to measure leg length.

If LLD exceeds 1 centimeter, the individual begins to compensate in other ways (long leg flexion, vaulting, circumduction, pelvic obliquity, and so on) in an effort to maintain energy efficiency. These compensations may have their own long-term consequences. With this degree of discrepancy, treatment to equalize the leg lengths should be undertaken. A shoelift is one possibility. If the discrepancy is detected prior to skeletal maturity a relatively simple percutaneous surgical epiphyseodesis of the long leg is done at an appropriate age. Once skeletal maturity has been reached, correction is more difficult requiring either shortening of the long leg or lengthening of the short leg. Each has its own unique problems, but I prefer not to shorten the patient's normal leg because of the potential severe consequences in the event of a complication. I have performed leg-lengthening procedures both acutely (in conjunction with a proximal femoral derotational osteotomy by incorporating valgus) and slowly over 4 to 8 weeks with an external fixator (such as the Ilizarov device). While this is possible, soft-tissue tightness problems require special attention during the lengthening process.

SCOLIOSIS

Scoliosis occurs in about one-third of individuals with hemiplegia. It is less common than in quadriplegia, but more frequent than idiopathic scoliosis (Koop et al. 1991). Surgery is seldom necessary. Occasionally a spinal deformity noted on an upright standing radiograph is due to lower extremity deformity, poor balance, or LLD. A sitting X-ray can help sort out some of these issues. Orthotic intervention in small or moderate curves can be effective in avoiding the need for surgical intervention. The spine is an important site of compensation to maintain the center of mass in an appropriate position within the base of support. Occasionally lumbopelvic motion is used to aid in forward progression. Due to these concerns, all efforts to ensure that mobility and flexibility at the lumbosacral junction should be made if surgery is performed. Generally ambulatory individuals with hemiplegia do not have severe pelvic obliquity, spinal decompensation, or extension of large curvatures below L4 warrenting instrumentation and fusion below that level.

Conclusion

The above discussion is meant to portray the surgical and non-surgical management options that are currently available and used at the author's institution. There is no 'cookbook' correct answer for the many decisions that are made. It is not possible to create a table with a listing of specific indications for each surgical procedure that if followed, would lead to an optimal result. Unfortunately, the treatment of gait deviations due to CP is not that straightforward. In hemiplegia, the ability to classify according to the four subtypes does help to organize one's thinking about surgical intervention.

Hopefully this chapter provides some insight into the numerous dilemmas in the management of the patient with hemiplegic CP. Certainly it should be apparent that abnormalities at multiple levels must be evaluated. They can then be treated simultaneously to avoid the creation of other problems and the need for numerous interventions over the years of a child's life. As one can see, the decisions are based heavily on the results of dynamic gait analysis.

Using this tool to evaluate the results of treatment is an ongoing process. In addition, advances in gait-modeling techniques are rapidly gaining clinical application. Questions have been and will be answered about actual musculotendinous lengths during gait and the effects of surgery on their force-generating capability (Delp and Zajac 1992). Similar techniques will provide essential information to improve decision-making in order that outcomes are maximized.

Analysis of functional outcomes will provide a better assessment of the individual's level of function in the community. This will require assessment of the pretreatment condition as well as the posttreatment outcome. The use of a functional assessment tool will be essential. At Gillette Children's Specialty Healthcare, MN, USA, a functional mobility tool has been developed and is currently being used. Validity and reliability testing is ongoing. Correlation between a functional assessment tool and an analysis of energy consumption will provide new insight into the importance of individual gait deviations, their energy expenditure costs, and functional losses. The impact of surgical solutions on these increased costs are being assessed. It is through the combination of gait-analysis techniques, functional outcomes assessment, and gait modeling that further advances will be made in the treatment of hemiplegia and other types of ambulatory CP.

ACKNOWLEDGEMENTS

The author would like to acknowledge Mary Trost, Jean Stout RPT, and Joyce Phelps Trost RPT for their assistance with the preparation of this manuscript.

REFERENCES

Baker, L.D. (1956) A rational approach to the surgical needs of the cerebral palsy patient. *Journal of Bone and Joint Surgery*, **38A**, 313–323.

Bleck, E.E., Holstein, A. (1963) Iliopsoas tenotomy for spastic hip flexion deformities in cerebral palsy. Paper presented at *American Academy of Orthopaedic Surgeons*, Chicago, IL, USA.

Bruce, R.W., Stout, J., Gage, J.R. (1994) Joint Kinetics in spastic hemiplegia. *Developmental Medicine and Child Neurology,* **(Suppl 90)**, 8–9.

Chung, C.Y., Stout, J., Gage, J.R. (1997) Rectus femoris transfer-gracilis vs. sartorius. *Gait and Posture*, **6,** 137–146.

Cosgrove, A.P., Corry, I.S., Graham, H.K. (May 1994) Botulinum toxin in the management of the lower limb in cerebral palsy. *Developmental Medicine and Child Neurology,* **36,** 386–396.

Delp, S.L., Zajac, F.E. (1992) Force- and moment-generating capacity of lower-extremity muscle before and after tendon lengthening. *Clinical Orthopedics and Related Research,* **284,** 247–259.

Dwyer, F.C. (1959) Osteotomy of the calcaneum for pes cavus. *Journal of Bone and Joint Surgery*, **41B,** 80.

Eggers, G.W.N. (1952) Transplantation of hamstring tendons to femoral condyles in order to improve hip extension and to decrease knee flexion in cerebral spastic paralysis. *Journal of Bone and Joint Surgery,* **34A,** 827–830.

Frost, H.M. (1971) Surgical treatment of spastic equinus in cerebral palsy. *Archives of Physical Medicine and Rehabilitation,* **52,** 270.

Gage, J.R. (1991) *Gait Analysis in Cerebral Palsy. Clinics in Developmental Medicine, No 121.* London: Mac Keith Press.

— Perry, J., Hicks, R.R., Koop, S., Werntz, J.R. (1987) Rectus femoris transfer as a means of improving knee function in cerebral palsy. *Developmental Medicine and Child Neurology*, **29,** 159–166.

Graham, H.K. (1995) Management of spasticity associated with cerebral palsy. *In:* O'Brien, C., Yablon, S. (Eds.) *Management of Spasticity with Botulinum Toxin.* Littleton, CO: Postgraduate Institute for Medicine, p. 17–23.

Green, N.E. (1992) Split posterior tibial tendon transfer: The universal procedure. *In:* Sussman, M.D. (Ed.) *The Diplegic Child.* Portland, OR: American Academy of Orthopedic Surgeons, p. 417–426.

Hiroshima, K., Hamada, S., Shimizu, N., Ohshita, S., Ono, K. (1988) Anterior transfer of the long toe flexors for the treatment of spastic equinovarus and equinus foot in cerebral palsy. *Journal of Pediatric Orthopaedics*, **8,** 164–8.

Hoffinger, S.A., Rab, G.T., Abou-Ghaida, H. (1993) Hamstrings in cerebral palsy crouch gait. *Journal of Pediatric Orthopaedics,* **13,** 722–726.

Kling, T.F. Jr, Schmidt, T.L., Conklin, J.J. (1991) Open wedge osteotomy of the first cuneiform for metatarsus adductus. Orthopaedic Transactions **15,** 106.

Koop, S.E., Lonstein, J.E., Winter, R.B., Denis, F. (1991) The natural history of spine deformity in cerebral palsy. Paper presented at the Scoliosis Research Society meeting, Minneapolis, MN, September, p. 209–210.

Novacheck, T.F. (1996) Surgical intervention in ambulatory cerebral palsy. *In:* Harris, G.F., Smith, P.A., (Eds.) *Human Motion Analysis.* Piscataway, NJ: IEEE Press, pp. 231–252.

— Chung, C.Y., Trost, J.P., Gage, J.R. (1996) Crouch gait in cerebral palsy-The effects of psoas lengthening. Paper presented at Pediatric Orthopaedic Society of North America, Phoenix, AZ, 15 May 1996, pp. 96.

O'Brien, C. (1995) Clinical pharmacology of botulinum toxin. *In:* O'Brien, C., Yablon, S. (Eds.) *Management of Spasticity with Botulinum Toxin.* Littleton, CO: Postgraduate Institute for Medicine, p. 3–6.

Õunpuu, S., Muik, E., Davis III, R.B., Gage, J.R., DeLuca, P.A. (1993a) Rectus femoris surgery in children with cerebral palsy. Part I: The effect of rectus femoris transfer location on knee motion. *Journal of Pediatric Orthopaedics,* **13,** 325–330.

— — — — — (1993b) Rectus femoris surgery in children with cerebral palsy. Part II: A comparison between the effect of transfer and release of the distal rectus femoris on knee motion. *Journal of Pediatric Orthopaedics,* **13,** 331–335.

111

Perry, J., Giovan, P., Harris, L.J., Montgomery, R.P.T., Azaria, M. (1978) The determinate of muscle action in the hemiparetic lower extremity and their effect on the examination procedure. *Clinical Orthopaedics and Related Research,* **131,** 78–79.

Root, L., Siegal, T. 1980) Osteotomy of the hip in children: Posterior approach. *Journal of Bone and Joint Surgery,* **62-A,** 571–575.

Rose, S.A., DeLuca, P.A., Davis III, R.B., Õunpuu, S., Gage, J.R., (1993) Kinematic and kinetic evaluation of the ankle after lengthening of the gastrocnemius fascia in children with cerebral palsy. *Journal of Pediatric Orthopaedics,* **13,** 6, 727–732.

Strayer, L. (1950) Recession of the gastrocnemius. *Journal of Bone and Joint Surgery,* **32-A,** 3, 671–6.

Sutherland, D.H,. Santi, M., Abel, M.F. (1990) Treatment of stiff-knee gait in cerebral palsy; a comparison by gait analysis of distal rectus femoris transfer versus proximal rectus release. *Journal of Pediatric Orthopaedics,* **10,** 433–442.

Tachdjian, M.O. (1990) The foot and leg. *In:* Wickland, E.H. (Ed.) *Pediatric Orthopedics.* Philadelphia, PA: WB Saunders, p. 2691–2693.

Winters Jr. T.F., Gage, J.R., Hicks, R. (March 1987) Gait patterns in spastic hemiplegia in children and young adults. *Journal of Bone and Joint Surgery,* **69A,** 438.

Ziv, I., Blackburn, N., Rang, M., Koreska, J. (1984) Muscle growth in normal and spastic mice. *Developmental Medicine and Child Neurology,* **26,** 94–99.

9
NEUROLOGY OF THE UPPER LIMB

J. Keith Brown and E. Geoffrey Walsh

Hemiplegiain childhood is due to destruction of brain tissue and, like a stroke at the other extreme of life, is most commonly either at the level of cerebral cortex or basal ganglia and internal capsule. The clinical features follow the site but do not follow the extent of the lesion on imaging (Molteni et al. 1987). Imaging may show a bilateral lesion even though the clinical picture is a unilateral hemiplegia (Steinlin et al. 1993). The many causes and the different extent of the damage seen on imaging means that apart from the wide variations in the motor component – for example, degree of functional loss, dystonia or spasticity – there is also wide variation in the other effects of the brain damage in terms of epilepsy, learning disability, slow speech development, specific learning disorder and behaviour problems.

Anatomy of hand function

Sir Charles Bell (1833), the great anatomist, wrote,"The motion of the fingers do not merely result from the action of the large muscles which lie on the forearm – these are for the more powerful actions; but in the palm of the hand, and between the metacarpal bones, there are small muscles (lumbricals and interossei), which perform the finer motions, expanding the fingers and moving them in every direction, with great quickness and delicacy. These are the organs which give the hand the power of spinning, weaving, engraving; and they produce the quick motions of the musician's fingers, they are called by the anatomist fidicinales*" (pp. 106–107).

Anyone who has dissected a hand, or even perused anatomical drawings, will know that it is a structure of very considerable complexity. Studies of the muscles controlling the fingers have been reviewed by Friden and Lieber (1996), the fibres of the lumbricals are exceptional for they run for almost the whole length of the muscle. This arrangement allows them to exert an almost constant contractile force over a long range of fibre lengths, depending on the length of the flexor digitorum profundus.

Many writers have emphasised the role of the thumb in grasping, being able to be opposed to the fingers. An early writer (Lawrence 1866), after comparing the human hand with that of other animals, wrote "The great superiority of the human hand arises from the size and strength of the thumb, which can be brought into a state of opposition to the fingers, and is hence of the greatest use in enabling us to grasp spherical bodies, and take up any

---

Fidicen (Latin): a player of a stringed instrument.

object in the hand, in giving a firm hold on whatever we seize, in executing all the mechanical processes of the arts, in writing, drawing, cutting, in short, in a thousand offices, which occur every moment of our lives, and which either could not be accomplished at all, if the thumb were absent, or would require the concurrence of both hands, instead of being done by one only" (p.109).

The need for an opposing pincer grip is emphasised in reconstructive surgery in children with congenital phocomelias and lobster-claw anatomical deformities.

Neuroanatomy of hand function
THE CORTICOSPINAL TRACT
The pyramidal tract is only present in mammals – birds and lower vertebrates operate mainly on their basal ganglia as the highest motor centre since their movements usually involve proximal and axial musculature and are often stereotyped, repetitive and automatic with no precise distal learned movements.

The pyramidal tract is the name given to the direct pathway from motor cortex to the anterior horn cells of the spinal cord without any synapses in mid brain, brain stem or any higher level in the cord but in which 80% of the fibres decussate in the pyramids of the medulla (Walshe 1965). There is, however, a direct uncrossed pathway, which runs in the anterior part of the spinal cord – the anterior corticospinal path – larger on the right than the left, so that it is still possible for the ipsilateral cerebral cortex to produce movement of a limb. There is also a corticobulbar tract which subserves voluntary control of the bulbar muscles and speech which is neither spinal nor pyramidal but is included in this system (Brodal 1992).

Only a small proportion of the corticospinal tract actually arises from the large Betz cells of the precentral cortex i.e. Brodman area 4. Using retrograde degeneration after a lesion of the pyramidal tract in the cervical or brain-stem region, 80% of Betz cells degenerate. Forty percent of the Betz cells in a cluster in the motor cortex will project to a single motor-neurone pool in the spinal cord, each muscle having its own pool of anterior horn cells in a type of muscle nucleus (Mountcastle 1997). Single nerve-cell stimulation suggests that the cortex does know about muscles as well as movements and each single muscle has representation in the motor cortex (Rothwell 1994, Mountcastle 1997). Other fibres forming the corticospinal tract have their cell bodies of origin in a wide cortical area.

A circumscribed lesion of the motor cortex can be shown to cause secondary failure in development of the corticospinal pathway which can most easily be seen in the internal capsule and medullary pyramid. This is seen in a pathological specimen in Figures 9.1a and b but can also be readily seen on MRI and the clinical severity of the corticospinal loss correlates with the loss of function (Bouza et al. 1994)

Experimental lesions of the pyramidal tract
The pyramidal projection is mainly to hand and forearm, it is the only innervation of distal muscles. A lesion would, therefore, be expected to affect distal muscles of the hand with relative preservation of proximal power. Cortical stimulation of the corticospinal pathway produces the largest response in distal muscles. A lesion has negative effects in the sense of loss of power and skills in distal muscles and a positive effect in that loss of presynaptic

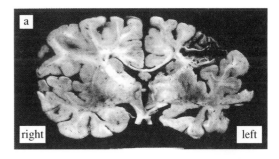

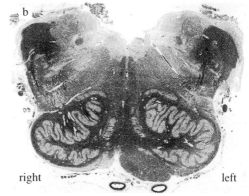

Fig. 9 1. *(a)* Small cortical infarct on the left with narrow internal capsule on same side. *(b)* Very poorly developed pyramid in medulla in same brain as *(a)*.

inhibition at the anterior horn cell causes increased excitability which is best demonstrated as brisk monosynaptic reflexes.

Sarah Towers (1940) made the first in-depth study of experimental pyramidal lesions in the cat in 1936 and in the monkey in 1940. There was loss of discrete use of the fingers with a grasp reflex, there was no visually directed placing, the whole arm was hooked round an object, there was loss of grasping and also withdrawl and the overriding posture was flexion of arm and leg. The monkeys could walk and run but were a little more flexed and adducted. Spasticity only occured if an additional lesion of the cerebral cortex was made in areas 4 and 6. The experiments of Tower were subsequently repeated by Twitchell and Denny-Brown (1966). Their findings were exactly the same.

A pyramidal lesion in man, therefore, might be expected to show the following deficits: (1) loss of fine individual digit movements, loss of reaching into space in the opposite hand and foot, loss of speed of movement of individual digits; (2) loss of learned voluntary skills i.e. a dyspraxia; (3) distal weakness (hemiparesis) with a 'cortical' wrist and foot drop and weak grasp – proximal 'windmill' or 'fly-swatting' movements are well preserved as is proximal power – ; (4) loss of segmental cord inhibition with release of monosynaptic reflexes, ankle clonus, and phasic, i.e. velocity-dependent, clasp-knife spasticity; (5) release of spinal flexor withdrawl reflex and also the return of a nociceptive Babinski sign with triple withdrawl.

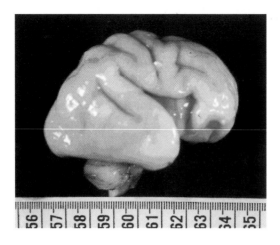

Fig. 9. 2. Brain of preterm infant showing hillocks on either side of central sulcus.

THE MOTOR CORTEX

The precentral gyrus, Brodman area 4, represents the primary motor area with its main outflow via the corticospinal tract. It appears first in the foetal brain as two distinct hillocks about 22 weeks' gestation and along with the calcarine sulci is the first cortical area to develop a distinct surface anatomical localisation (Fig. 9.2).

The motor strip has a thick cortex of about 4 mm and is distinguished histologically by the large Betz cells. The Betz cell, apart from its size, has abundant Nissl bodies and a large nucleolus and a large amount of active DNA, suggesting memory function. The dendrites of the Betz cells are in contact with neurones in all layers of the cortex. The motor cortex is organised into modules or the 'minicolumns' of Mountcastle (Mountcastle 1997) in a vertical direction as well as the classical horizontal six layers.

The precentral gyrus is the area which when stimulated at operation, as performed by Penfield and Rassmussen (1950) in humans, can be shown to result in movements of the opposite side of the body in a set order, i.e. the representation of the body as a homunculus. The representation of the body hanging by the foot from the top of the hemisphere along the central sulcus with the hand and face together as though the thumb was in the mouth is now well established not only from the study of pathology, stimulation and ablation but now by functional imaging. The segment of the precentral gyrus that most often contains motor hand function is a knob-like structure which corresponds precisely to the characteristic 'middle knee' of the central sulcus that was described by anatomists in the last century (Fig. 9.3) and is now confirmed by functional MRI (Yousry et al. 1997). PET studies have shown that sensory hand function is located in the post central region at the superior genu of the central sulcus (Rumeau et al. 1994). Each direction of movement may also have its own corresponding module. The motor cortex in the precentral gyrus is a kind of piano keyboard upon which the tunes stored in kinaesthetic memory can be played.

116

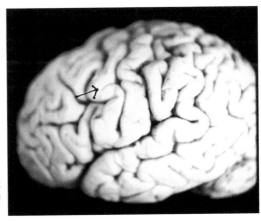

Fig. 9.3. Lateral surface of brain showing precentral gyrus with 'knee' at site of the hand in the motor cortex..

Motor association areas

Each part of the body represented by the homunculus has an association area ajacent to it. This area is responsible for storing the memories of learned skills i.e. an engram of movement sequences, so-called kinaesthetic memory. The hand association area contains the area for manual construction (constructional praxis) but also on the left for writing – the graphomotor area. The association area ajacent to the lips, tongue and palate contains Broca's area on the left for the learning of the motor sequences required for speech. In order to prevent interference from the opposite side by mirror movements and so allow a definite direction for a sequence of movements, the opposite modules in the corresponding hemisphere are inhibited (i.e. reciprocal cerebral inhibition or cerebral dominance). The more learned a skill the more lateralised it is and so likely to be lost in a unilateral cerebral lesion. Reorganisation of the cortical representation of the hand after damage in hemiplegia can also change the basic anatomy with the development of an ipsilateral association area for the hand (Carr 1996). In a recent study with patients with hemiparesis (Chollet et al. 1991) ipsilateral activation was found with movements of the affected hand.

Supplementary motor area

This lies in the frontal lobe on the medial surface, above the cingulate gyrus and anterior to the leg area of the motor strip. The supplementary motor area has a major input from the basal ganglia, such as the globus pallidus via the ventrolateral nucleus of the thalamus, which means it has all the information at its finger tips on body position and posture. It involves proximal (independent of the corticospinal pathway) as well as distal muscles (dependent upon the corticospinal pathway).

Stimulation of the supplementary motor area (SMA) produces movements of all four limbs bilaterally, trunk movement and vocalisation. It appears that, unlike the premotor cortex, only one side is needed and removal unilaterally does not produce motor impaiment. Stimulation produces complex bilateral sequences, movements and postures. Simple flexion–extension movements do not require the SMA but sequenced movements as in the

Denkla test of sequenced finger and thumb opposition or planning movements use the SMA. Bimanual activities are impaired in SMA lesions. The expression of emotion, cadence, intonation, hand gesture and facial expression, arising in the limbic and cingulate complex is also conducted via the supplementary motor area and via the extrapyramidal system.

Anticipation of an activity, such as planning a movement, is accompanied by electrical and metabolic activity in the SMA which can precede movement by as much as a second (Brooks 1986). It is sufficient to imagine or plan the movement in order to activate the supplementary motor area (Roland et al. 1980). Blood flow increases maximally when using several digits or joints and planning a complex sequence of movements (Roland et al. 1980). Using functional MRI Rao and colleagues (1995) have confirmed the findings of Roland, simple finger movements activate the contralateral primary motor cortex, whereas more complex movements activate the SMA bilaterally and also the contralateral somatosensory cortex. Therefore, the SMA and premotor cortex play an important role in the programming of complex sequenced motor acts (Catalan 1998). The SMA is selectively involved in imagining a complex motor act. A difference is also noted between right-handed people with strong left-hemisphere function and left-handed individuals who may have a right- or ipsilateral left-hemisphere dominance (Kim et al. 1993).

THE CEREBELLUM

Due to the vast amount of information which arrives at the brain from eyes, muscle spindles, tendon organs, labyrinths, proprioception and body contact, the cortex needs it to be presorted into subdepartments. There are loops from cortex to thalamus and back, to basal ganglia and back, and to cerebellum and back. The cerebellum has 40 times more input than output fibres and contains 50% of all neurones, yet in cerebellar disease there is no sensory loss. The cerebellum knows if we are standing or lying, our head position in relation to our body, position of limbs, and state of contraction of all muscles and their speed of contraction, tension produced and speed of shortening together with knowledge of extrapersonal space and distance of objects from the body. In normal function the basal ganglia and cerebellum probably send no output to the spinal cord and lower centres but all output is channelled back to the cortex via the cortical loop. It is thought that there is point-to-point somatotrophic representation between cerebral cortex and cerebellar cortex. The corticopontine fibres arise in the motor strip, SMA and somatosensory area (responsible for body image). The cortical projection passes via the internal capsule then the cerebral peduncle to the pons where they synapse in the nuclei pontis, cross to the opposite side and form the bridge of the pons and the middle cerebellar peduncle.

The information about a movement planned by the cortex is thus passed to the Purkinje cells. These have a vast arborisation of dendrites in contact with all the incoming sensory information. This is computed and the information is then sent back to the cerebral cortex. It helps the cortex to make the decision on what force, speed, direction and distance is required of the muscles to execute the planned movement most smoothly.

Incoordination or ataxia is the name given to the clumsiness of movements which occurs when we use too much force and break an object, too little force and drop it, or misjudge distance and knock it over. We classify these as neurological signs of dysmetria, intention tremor, past pointing and clumsiness. These signs are the most obvious abnormality in the adult but in the child the disruption of motor learning causes slow development of speech rather than the explosive, staccato, slurred dysarthria of the adult and the disruption of motor learning in the hand may resemble a dyspraxia rather than simple incoordination. The main functions of the cerebellum can be summarised as follows: to stabilise the body and limb during a movement, to set speed, force, distance, direction, and to provide a motor memory for repeated stereotyped actions, i.e. learned skills.

Cerebellum and spasticity
The output from the Purkinje cells is driven by the ring circuit from the motor cortex. If the input from the cortex is lost due to cerebral cortical damage then the Purkinje inhibition of the cerebellar nuclei is absent and they can respond directly to incoming stimuli such as that from the muscle spindles via the dorsal spinocerebellar tract (Fig. 9.4). This is the basis of 'tonic spasticity'. If the cerebellum is removed then the reverse ('tonic paresis') occurs with hypotonia as seen in a hypotonic ataxic diplegia. It is, therefore, a normal cerebellum in the presence of an abnormal cerebral cortex which causes spasticity and an abnormal cerebellum with a normal cortex which causes hypotonia.

Basal ganglia and hand skills
The basal ganglia like the cerebellum have a loop system with the cerebral cortex. They are regarded as extrapyramidal as they affect muscles through a different pathway than the corticospinal pathway and allow two messages at once to be sent to a group of muscles. The expression of emotion in the right hemisphere can, therefore, be superimposed upon the logical thoughts of language from the left. In this way intonation is imposed upon speech, sprightliness on gait or on hand gesture, and stress for expression of feeling on a hand skill such as playing the piano.

We shall not consider the basal ganglia in detail as this part of the motor circuit has mainly to do with posture, gait and expression of emotion although it can have an effect on hand skills or swinging the arms when walking. The cadence of actions such as the speed of speech, speed of writing and elective walking speed are determined by this system. If the basal ganglia are damaged then stiffness in muscles together with the difficulty starting a movement – bradykinesia – means all movements including writing are slow and of small amplitude, such as in micrographia.

The importance of the basal ganglia in hemiplegia is when abnormal tone, i.e. dystonia, imposes a posture as a hemiplegic posture, dystonia or athetosis which may completely disrupt the attempts of the pyramidal system to perform any skilled movement. Involuntary movements such as tremor, tics, chorea or myoclonus may be released in basal ganglia disease and can then further disrupt voluntary movements.

CONCLUSION
The reason for giving this brief review of neuroanatomy is to give an explanation as to why we see a weak hemiplegia, a dyspraxic hemiplegia, a spastic hemiplegia, a hypotonic hemiplegia, a dystonic hemiplegia, a hemiplegia with ataxia or a hemiplegia with athetosis.

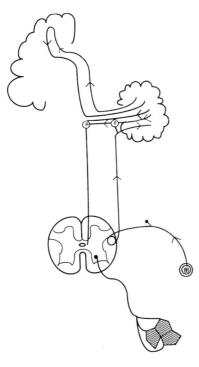

Fig. 9.4. Relation of the corticocerebellar and spinocerebellar pathways in spasticity.

The posture of the limb, the muscle tone, reflex changes, the distal weakness and loss of skills may all appear independent of each other. This depends upon the site of damage whether it be cortex, basal ganglia, cortex without cerebellum, cortex with cerebellum or corticospinal tract alone. A hemiplegia is not a uniform neurological abnormality but a syndrome not only due to many causes but with many clinical components so that there is a wide variation in the clinical signs between different patients.

Normal maturation of hand function

At birth, hand control is purely reflex so that an object placed in the palm of the hand and to which traction is applied results in a firm grasp reflex. If the dorsum of the hand is stimulated or if the arm is extended and the back of the hand placed against the buttock the hand opens and remains open allowing the inspection of the palm. The hand also opens with the Moro reflex but if a grasp reflex is initially elicited it inhibits the Moro on that side. One hand closes and the opposite opens as part of an asymmetrical tonic neck reflex. The hand and mouth tend to mirror each other in that they open together.

By 4 weeks past term the flexor tone in the arms has been inhibited. The traction response is less although the grasp reflex will stay until the age of 3 months. From around 3 months the child develops hand regard and looks at her/his hands while moving them in front of her/his face. In individuals with severe learning disability this may persist. Forced grasping by pulling at the clothes, and sometimes the knitting movements which return in Rett syndrome may be seen in the normally developing infant at this stage. Voluntary release of an object placed in her/his hand is the first sign of volition in the development of hand function and occurs as the obligatory grasp reflex is inhibited.

By 4 months of age the grasp reflex is completely inhibited unless the hand is placed at the side of the ear and traction of the grasped object applied. It is thought that inhibition of the grasp reflex is controlled by the motor areas of the frontal lobe. The grasp reflex will return if there is pathology of the frontal lobe, i.e. tumours, strokes or in acute head injuries. As the grasp reflex disappears voluntary opening and closing of the hands appears so that by 5 months the infant can reach out for an object, grasp it, move it towards her/his head, hit her/his face and then by using the rooting reflex get an object into her/his mouth. He simply moves her/his hand in the direction of the object until s/he hits the object and grasps it. At this stage the infant's coordination maturation is poor. S/he has no idea of distance and pushes an object too far into her/his mouth and gags. To an adult neurologist all normal infants would be considered to have signs of cerebellar disease. By 6 months the hands are in the midline and the child is able to pass objects from one hand to the other. Objects can be placed in the mouth without using the rooting reflex which has now been inhibited and the distance to which an object is placed in the mouth is more finely regulated.

GRASPS

Early grasping consists of crude palming movements in which the three ulnar fingers predominate whereas the thumb is practically inactive. By about 10 months of age, this grasp is succeeded by a refined finger prehension characterised principally by thumb opposition, forefinger dominance and adaptation of finger pressure to the weight of the object. Grasping is often divided into two main subdivisions – power grasps and precision grasps. In the precision grasp the hand starts to open and the fingers form the most approriate shape for the object, under visual guidance, early in the reaching process and before the hand hits the object (Forssberg 1998). When a child sees an object which s/he wants to grasp s/he has to make several very sophisticated decisions which depend upon anticipation of the characteristics of the object from previous, i.e. learned, experience (Thelen and Ronnqvist 1988): (1) does the task require one or two hands? Infants of 6 months can decide this by assessing the size of the object before hand contact. (2) How many fingers need to be opposed to the thumb – one (pincer), two (pencil), three fingers (cone) or all four fingers for around the top of a glass or container, for example. (3) All fingers to palm i.e. palmar grasp or dagger or the power grasp for squeezing which again is decided before hand contact by the appearance and size of the object. (4) All fingers and thumb extended and abducted to object with no opposition (e.g. to hold the top of a large container)

Which type of grip is required is largely determined by vision, i.e. it is a visuomotor skill. One also has to determine the force or power required and this is probably proprioception dependent upon the feeling of slippage of the object. Just as there is a dictionary of grasps so also there is a dictionary of basic manipulations: (1) lift (at wrist, elbow or shoulder), (2) push, (3) shake (up and down at wrist), (4) screw (pronation and supination), (5) circle (at wrist with flexion, extension, pronation, supination).

Therefore, the infant has to develop two basic mechanisms, i.e. pinch and lift. At first these are independent but eventually, before the age of 2 years, they merge into a smooth synergistic movement. Grip is initially tighter than required for the task so the force is higher in infants than in older children. Initially on contact with an object one grips and then lifts monitoring the forces required to prevent slip. A slippery object requires more grip force to prevent slip even though lift force need be no greater (Forssberg 1998). Adults adjust their grip to 50% above slip which is then held constant and stable, but young children overcompensate by 300%. Both these tasks of judging force and synergism would be expected to be manifestations of cerebellar maturation as described above.

REACHING
Reaching is obviously dependent upon the development of something more than neuromuscular activity requiring the coordination of visual and motor mechanisms. By the time the infant is beginning to reach, at about 4 months old, s/he has definite cortical vision and can recognise parents, food, favourite toys and so on. The arms may wave in the direction of an object in younger infants but the object acts as an alerting response and triggers innate doggy paddling movements. Martin Bax pointed out (personal communication) one should not cover the legs when examining an infant and one could then see the similiar movements in the legs. Normally the first reaching movements occur in the supine position. When a rattle is held 4 inches above an infant's chest s/he looks at it only momentarily during the first 8 weeks. From 8 to 12 weeks s/he makes small incipient movements with transient regard of the object and the arm activity is increased. Visually directed reaching is one of the most striking developments during the first 6 months and it marks an important step towards the mastery of objects and tools. Between the age of 22 and 30 postnatal weeks, the movements become considerably slower, and predominantly single handed. By the age of 32 and 52 weeks, reaching is dramatically stabilised with the return of bimanual activity (Thelen et al. 1993).

The movement of the arm in reaching involves major adjustment of other parts of the body to prevent toppling over due to altering the position of the body's centre of gravity. The elevation of both arms effects a change in a preexisting posture and must be counterbalanced by readjustments of the body in relation to the supporting surface and the force of gravity. At first the infant cannot reach and sit and needs supported sitting to free the hands. If balance is poor then tripod sitting may prevent all use of the hands.

Body image and extrapersonal space
If one is not aware of the sensation that one has a limb then it may be neglected and not used even though it is not paralysed. Equally, with phantom-limb syndrome one may try to use a limb which no longer exists. Lost or impaired body image is often incriminated as the cause of poor motor performance in children with cerebral palsy (CP). When artificial limbs were tried in children with phocomelia from thalidomide embryopathy it was often extremely frustrating that children did not seem to use mechanically ingenious artificial limbs and could not incorporate them into their body image. Instead they would use their feet with great dexterity, learning sophisticated skills such as using a knife and fork, peeling an apple or

threading a needle. It is the motor learning in the brain and not the anatomy which is the most important.

Body image and sense of extrapersonal space are developed through sensory feedback from the body's senses of touch and pressure which feed through the thalamus to the primary sensory cortex and the vision of self and others which projects to the calcarine cortex and then the visual association areas. These unite in the posterior parietal cortex to give the sense of shape of objects, extrapersonal space, direction and body image. The child in the second year of life identifies gradually more parts of the body on her/himself and her/his parents. Children with hemiplegia will sometimes draw a human figure with one arm missing.

Animals whose arms are splinted with cardboard tubes during early development will be poorer at manipulative skills. Exploratory behaviour, both visual and tactile, gives the child a concept of objects that have size, shape, weight, temperature and texture, that is a kind of object language so that anticipation of the force, speed, distance the limb has to travel and the type of grasp most appropriate eventually becomes automatic.

Clinical features of congenital hemiplegia

In our patients males outnumber females – of 100 subjects with congenital hemiplegia there were 62 males and 38 females. Right-sided hemiplegia was twice as common as left-sided hemiplegia in congenital cases: right 70%, left 30%, but this preponderance of lateralisation does not apply in acquired cases. The preponderance of right-sided hemiplegia applies to both males and females with congenital hemiplegia, but there is a suggestion that with changes in neonatology there is an increasing preponderance of left-sided hemiplegia.

EARLY DIAGNOSIS OF HEMIPLEGIA

Neonatal period

All neonates have brisk tendon reflexes, ankle clonus, crossed reflexes, reflex hand opening, increased flexor muscle tone, no voluntary reaching or independent finger control, i.e. they all have a bilateral hemiplegia by adult neurological criteria. A perinatal stroke may have occurred weeks before birth but may be symptomatically silent or present only as fits in an otherwise normally developing infant. Such infants may show symmetrical movements, equal flexor tone, symmetrical grasp reflexes and symmetrical tendon reflexes even in the presence of a gross cortical lesion. A hemisyndrome is not the same as a hemiplegia and may in fact appear on the opposite side from a future hemiplegia. Early diagnosis before 3 months of age is difficult as an asymmetry does not mean a future hemiplegia and an absence of asymmetry does not rule out a severe hemiplegia.

A hemisyndrome may be of three types:

(1) Paralytic – when there is weakness with poverty of movement or inability to support the weight on that side using reflexes, this is often due to cervical cord, or brachial plexus lesions (brought about by trauma, myelodysplasia, neuroblastoma, neonatal polyneuritis, for example). Spontaneous doggy paddling or cycling movements may be absent unilaterally following asphyxia.

(2) A reflex hemisyndrome may be seen during recovery from asphyxia and can affect either phasic reflexes such as asymmetrical tendon reflexes, ankle clonus or postural reflexes

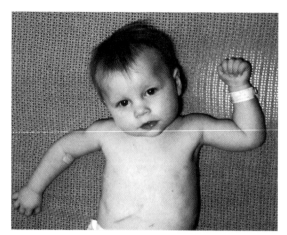

Fig. 9.5. Fisted and externally rotated hemiplegic arm.

such as the Moro, asymmetrical tone neck reflex crossed-extension or trunk-incurvation reflexes or may be associated with asymmetric movements and tone.

(3) The third type of hemisyndrome is asymmetrical muscle tone usually consisting of extensor hypertonus on one side, with relative hypotonia on the other so that recoil, scarf signs, popliteal angles and range of dorsiflexion are asymmetrical.

Early postnatal development
In a child with hemiplegia the movement of the upper limbs becomes more asymmetrical by 4 months of age with a lessening of movement on the affected side. The hand on the affected side tends to lie abducted at the side of the head and does not develop the normal internal rotation with the hand in the midline (Fig. 9.5). At 3 months', the normally developing child starts to look at her/his hands (hand regard) and to reach out and pull at her/his clothes (forced grasping), both of these in the infant with hemiplegia will be reduced on the affected side. Although s/he will hold an object placed in her/his hands, using the grasp reflex, s/he cannot release it on the affected side. The hand appears to remain tightly closed with the fingers closed over the thumb which is adducted across the palm. A hemiplegia may be wrongly suspected in a normally developing infant as the hands do not mature at identical speeds so the grasp may disappear in the left hand before the right hand (Fig. 9.6). This is in keeping with the greater blood flow to the right hemisphere up to 3 years of age (Chiron 1997).

At 5 months of age the child with hemiplegia fails to reach, hold an object,or get an object to her/his mouth using the affected side. There will usually be no spasticity at this stage. Since ankle clonus is normal in some infants up to 4 months' its absence or presence is not significant and the infant with hemiplegia will stand with feet flat even though later the leg may be severely spastic with an equinus deformity.

By 6 months' the arm will be obviously abnormal with failure of development of manipulative skills but it may be thought to be a monoplegia and even careful examination

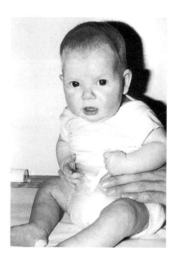

Fig. 9.6. Fisted left hand with inhibition of grasp reflex on the right.

at this stage may reveal little neurological abnormality in the leg. In the arm, parachute responses do not develop (Fig. 9.7) and spasticity of the pronators appears. In the leg spasticity and a tendency to equinus appear in the second half of the first year. Some have suggested a scoring system for abnormal motor patterns as an aid to early diagnosis (Morgan 1996).

THE ESTABLISHED HEMIPLEGIA
Components of a hemiplegia
In the older child with an established hemiplegia there is marked variation in the clinical findings from case to case. This is because the pattern of actual brain damage differs in site and severity. The various components which may form the hemiplegia 'constellation' are listed below and will now be considered in more detail.
• Weak grasp
• Loss of fine sequenced movement of the fingers
• Retention of proximal power – 'fly swatting'
• Loss of speed of movements
• Retention of grasp reflex
• Loss of fine motor skills (dyspraxia)
• Associated and mirror movements
• Wrist drop
• Spasticity of long finger flexors, thumb adductor and biceps
• Flexed, internally rotated limb
• Athetoid posturing
• Dystonic flexion or extension
• Absent protective reflexes
• Brisk tendon reflexes
• Cold blue feet with delayed capillary return

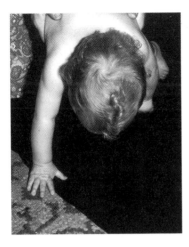

Fig. 9.7. Asymmetrical parachute response with failure to develop on the left.

- Smaller nails
- Short thin limb: trophic change
- Delayed bone age
- Loss of sensation
- Inability to wiggle toes
- Foot drop – weak dorsiflexors
- Equinus on passive dorsiflexion
- Equinus on active dorsiflexion
- Toe grasp in extrapyramidal hemiplegia
- Loss of speed at toes, ankle and in acceleration at the hip
- Leg extended, internally rotated, weight bearing
- Spasticity of calf, hamstrings and adductors
- Clasp-knife response to rapid stretch
- No spasticity of midline muscles i.e. jaw, trunk or hip
- Brisk tendon reflexes
- Ankle clonus
- Extensor Babinski sign to nociceptive stimulus
- Dynamic internal rotation at end swing if dystonic
- All individuals with hemiplegia will walk unless precluded by associated disabilities
- Decrease in maximum walking speed
- Leg on affected side accelerates more slowly
- Loss of terminal knee extension in swing
- Toe strike, toe – heel– back knee or side foot strike

PARESIS AND WEAKNESS OF MOVEMENT
Hemiparesis is taken to mean weakness of one side of the body and hemiplegia as complete paralysis. It is rare to lose all proximal movement except in the acute stage of a stroke but

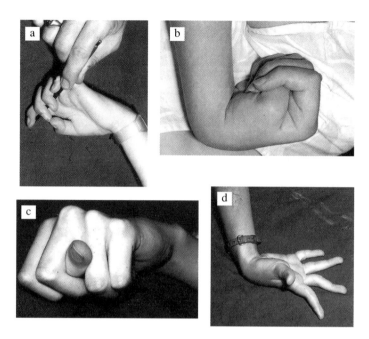

Fig. 9.8. *(a)* Flexion of fingers and adduction of thumb with traction on fingers. *(b)* Flexed wrist, adducted thumb over tightly flexed fingers in a hemiplegic hand. *(c)* Grasp reflex retained with the 'mana obscena' position. *(d)* Secondary subluxation of the metacarpophalangeal joint of the thumb and interphalangeal joints of the fingers.

in children with hemiplegia proximal power is nearly always well preserved even in the presence of a hand that is totally immobile. Proximal muscle movements are preserved so that fly swatting or 'windmill' movements of the affected arm may be well performed. The arm is often cited as being more affected than the leg but the arm is used for fast fine independent distal digital movements and the leg for the better preserved proximal gross movements used in walking. The hand will always cause some manipulative difficulty yet 100% of children with hemiplegic CP should walk unless precluded by associated disabilities.

The hand is kept closed and there is a retained grasp reflex, at a maximum when a pen or similar object is placed in the hand and traction applied to it especially with the arm flexed at the elbow and the child lying with the hand at the side of the head (Fig. 9.8a). If the position of the arm is reversed and the limb is extended and internally rotated with the back of the hand on the buttock, the hand opens and the grasp is released and traction no longer causes finger flexion. The adductor pollicis muscle is usually very spastic so the thumb is kept adducted across the palm inside the fisted hand (Fig. 9.8b) and may protrude between the second and third fingers as the so-called mana obscena (Fig. 9.8c). In order to voluntarily abduct the thumb the metacarpophalangeal joint is often dislocated so that the phalangeal part of the thumb abducts while its metacarpal stays adducted (Fig. 9.8d). The fingers themselves

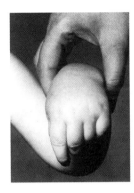

Fig. 9.9. Wrist drop as part of the hemiplegic posture due to weak wrist extensors.

extend at the metacarpophalangeal joints and flex at the interphalangeal. There is no pincer grasp, fine individual finger movements are lost and the child cannot oppose each finger and thumb in turn. The child can no more wiggle the toes than s/he can her/his fingers. There is a wrist drop and a foot drop due to peripheral selective extensor weakness (Fig. 9.9).

Weakness of movement is not a total paralysis in the sense of a lower motor neurone lesion but a loss of volitional sequenced distal skilled movements. These weak voluntary muscles will still contract strongly as part of the grasp reflex, spastic stretch response or finger jerk. It may still be possible to activate individual motor units by using mirror movement from the opposite limb. Mirror movements may be very marked from good to bad hand but may occur in the opposite direction up to the age of 10 years (Nass 1985). A very sensitive test for minor degrees of distal weakness is the inability to touch each finger in turn to the thumb – the Denckla test (Denckla 1973). Even sequential finger movements such as in the Denckla test can be made as mirror movements.

Voluntary grasp is measured by squeezing the examiner's fingers, by forcibly opposing the thumb and index finger while the examiner tries to pull her/his finger between them, more objectively by dynamometry or by clinical MRC grading. The voluntary grasp on the hemiplegic side is very significantly weak compared to the unaffected side $p = 0.0001$ (Fig. 9.10 a, b) (Brown et al. 1987). Using a grip dynamometer it can be shown that grip strength on the unaffected side increases with age (5 to 15 years) from 3 to 15 pounds per square inch but not on the hemiplegic side. The functional use of the hand is strongly correlated to the loss of distal power (see below).

Even in severe cases with loss of function of individual finger movements there may be good recruitment of isolated motor units when attempting a graded control of finger pressure on a lever monitored by EMG feedback (Harrison and Connolly 1971). Children with CP have much more difficulty in adjusting fingertip pressure and anticipating the characteristics of an object. Normally developing children achieve adult levels of fingertip force adjustment by 7 to 8 years but children with CP only have the force adjustment of a normal 1 year old by this age (Eliasson et al. 1991, Gordon and Forssberg 1997). They require multiple trials with the hemiplegic hand to anticipate the lift/force required for an object but if allowed to use the unaffected hand first of all the internal sensory image, or object concept, is built up more

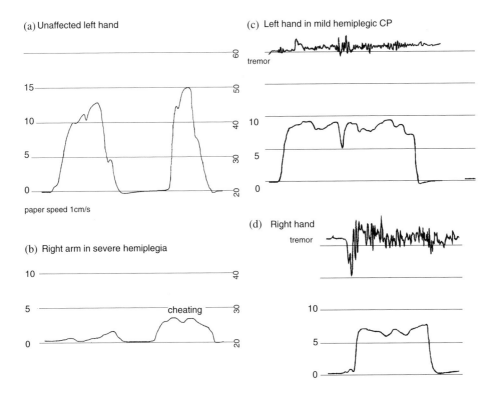

Fig. 9.10. *(a)* Apparently normal left hand in a child with right-sided hemiplegia. The force of a squeeze is indicated.*(b)* The affected right side of the same patient. The squeeze is weak. *(c)* Left hand in a child with mild hemiplegic CP. The power is reasonably good and sustained, the top trace is a record of tremor which is only mild. *(d)* Right hand on the affected side of another child but with more severe hemiplegia. The power is fairly poor and the tremor associated with the action is substantial. Units of calibration lines pounds per square inch power.

rapidly and the child is better able to use the hemiplegic hand (Gordon and Duff 1999)

One of us (EGW) has measured the accuracy with which two fingers can be moved synchronously in students and older people without CP (Walsh 1997). The timing when two fingers made or broke contact with Morse keys or with electrical conductors was measured (Fig. 9.11). When the discs were used most individuals showed some 'overlap', one finger being fully flexed before the other started to be extended and the person with minimal CP showed great slowness when trying to extend one finger while flexing the other, a 'contrary' movement. This person did comparatively well when flexing or extending two fingers at the same time. Children, and particularly boys, found it very difficult to perform the test where two fingers are required to move in opposite directions at the same time (unpublished work of Milling-Smith et al.).

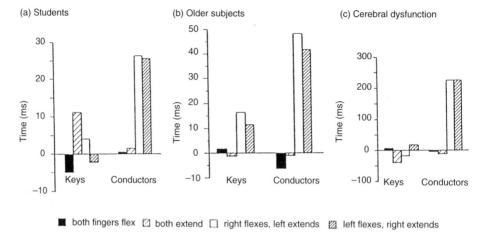

(a) Students   (b) Older subjects   (c) Cerebral dysfunction

■ both fingers flex ▨ both extend □ right flexes, left extends ▨ left flexes, right extends

Fig 9.11. *(a)* Movements of left and right index fingers of students. There were differences for the contrary movements with keys or conductive discs; with the discs there was overlap. *(b)* Results with older persons are broadly similar. *(c)* A person with minimal cerebral dysfunction. For antiphase movements there were long delays in extending the appropriate finger when using the discs. Note that the vertical scales of the diagrams are different (Walsh 1997).

SPEED OF MOVEMENT

This depends upon maturation of the corticospinal pathway, and it also depends upon the mechanical speed at which muscle can contract. There is a greater physiological stiffness of muscles in the younger child, a kind of developmental myotonia, which lessens with age allowing speed to increase. This is, however, counteracted by more inertia as the length of the limb increases (Walsh and Wright 1987, Lin et al. 1996). Also, at a certain threshold speed there is a fusion response (fusion frequency), for example, the fingers stop moving at a certain speed and movement transfers to the wrist. Using the Jebsen hand-function test in acquired hemiplegia both hands are found to be slower than normal but in left hemiplegia movement is slower than in right (Spaulding et al. 1988) – a finding which we verified in children (Brown et al. 1987). The speed of finger movements can be measured by finger-to-thumb opposition, repeated opposition of thumb to other fingers in sequence which can be timed as the number of oppositions in 10 seconds, tapping with a pencil, making dots, moving pegs in a peg board or by physiological measurements with an accelerometer on the finger. The normal maximum speed of fast tapping is around 6 per second. Loss of speed of movement is the most sensitive indicator of the severity of a hemiplegia and the hemiplegic hand is significantly slower than the good hand ($p=0.0001$). Like distal weakness the loss of speed has a strong correlation with the loss of function of the limb (see below) (Brown et al. 1987).

LOSS OF LEARNED HAND SKILLS.

Motor learning requires concentration (attention), consciousness (alertness), motivation (application), and practice (repetition) (Regan and Brown 1998). Motor skills are not cognitive

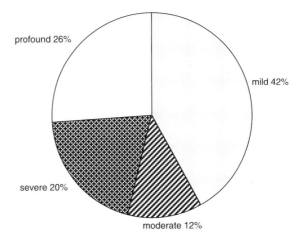

Fig. 9.12. Pie chart showing the percentage loss of function in the affected compared to the unaffected hand in 50 children with hemiplegia.

profound 26%

mild 42%

severe 20%

moderate 12%

and so do not depend upon a symbol system or language but depend on memorising and practising a sequenced movement pattern, that is on kinaesthetic memory. This has been supported by the demonstration of the arrest of cognitive learning but preservation of motor learning after anterior temporal lobectomy. The opposite is also true. That is to say, a child can have a normal IQ and yet have the hand skills of a much younger child (Minns et al. 1977).

Observation of a surgeon, skilled typist, keyboard operator or a violinist will confirm that, with training, great versatility of control, precision and increased speed of a learned skill can be achieved (Poore 1873). A dyspraxia relates to the inability to learn how to perform a motor skill which is commensurate with the child's age. This may involve hand manipulation with a constructional dyspraxia, writing as a dyspraxic dysgraphia, a dressing dyspraxia, gross postural skills in a gymnastic dyspraxia, or speech in an articulatory dyspraxia. In a pure genetic dyspraxia there is no associated distal weakness, spasticity, change in reflexes, incoordination, abnormal posture: simple repetitive movements can be performed but cannot be sequenced into a skill.

The ability to slot Lego together, take a sweet out of its paper, pour juice from a jug, build with blocks, cut with scissors, use a knife and fork, tie shoe laces, catch a ball in one hand, thread a needle and so on is developed in a specific sequence. Although some IQ tests have components testing motor skills, such as folding a piece of paper or cutting with scissors, they may miss children with very severe developmental dyspraxia. A standardised test of hand function is necessary. The imitation of gestures; miming how an object in a picture is used; the copying of manipulation of levers on a board according to pictures; the manipulation in three-dimensional space of grommets on a wire or of actual tools can all form the basis of a formal hand-function test. An attempt to provide normative data for hand function has been developed by O'Hare (1998 personal communication). This allows us to construct tests of hand manipulative skills.

When measuring such skills, difficulty arises because experience and the amount of previous practice vary enormously. Skills such as changing a plug, typing, playing a musical

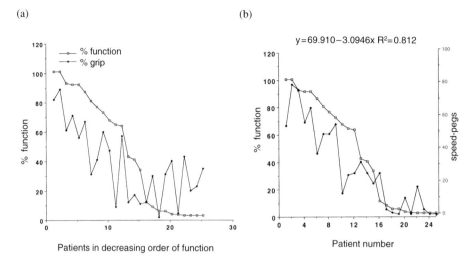

(a)   (b)

$y=69.910-3.0946x \; R^2=0.812$

Patients in decreasing order of function

Patient number

Fig. 9.13. *(a)* Very close relation of function in a hemiplegic hand to loss of distal power. *(b)* Close relation of loss of function in the hemiplegic hand with poor performance in speed tests.

instrument or even playing computer games will all depend upon the amount of practice an individual has had. Speed measurements are necessary in normally developing older children which obviously poses an unfair penalty for children with neurological disabilities.

Severity of functional loss will range from very mild to very severe. The easiest way to gauge severity in children with hemiplegia is to compare good and bad hand function in some form of standardised test. In 50 children examined in this way (Fig. 9.12) 42% were classified as mild (hemiplegic hand 75% function compared with good hand), 12% as moderate (50 to 75% function), 20% severe (25 to 50% function) and 26% very severe (less than 25% ability in the affected compared to the unaffected hand). The left hand also appears to experience greater functional loss when hemiplegic than the right hand. We can now compare the degree of functional loss with the other neurological findings. We find a very strong correlation with loss of speed and loss of distal power (Fig. 9.13a, b).

ABNORMALITIES OF MUSCLE TONE

Children with CP have limbs which feel stiff and offer increased resistance on attempts to move their joints. To many clinicians all stiffness is described as spasticity and they feel there is little to be gained clinically by trying to subdivide this into phasic spasticity, tonic spasticity, rigidity, plasticity, thixotropy, or short muscle disease (Brown and Minns 1989). This is not now acceptable as treatments such as intramuscular botulinum toxin, intrathecal baclofen or selective dorsal rhizotomy may help certain types of stiffness and not others.

Muscle tone can be simply defined as the resistance felt when a limb is passively rotated about a joint. The factors contributing to this resistance can be divided into those due to joints,

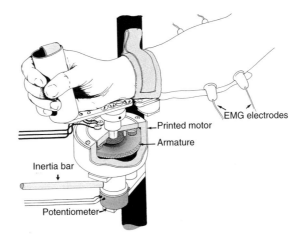

Fig. 9.14. Diagram to illustrate the attachment of the hand to a torque generator motor.

EMG electrodes

Printed motor

Armature

Inertia bar

Potentiometer

ligaments and soft tissues and those due to muscle itself. This resistance from muscle can be divided into three components: (1) electrical contraction – tension or failure to relax, phasic spasticity, tonic spasticity and rigidity; (2) non-electrical biomechanical resistance of muscle and tendon – viscosity, elasticity, plasticity, thixotropy; (3) resistance which is in some cases electrically active and in some electrically silent such as cramp, tetany and myotonia.

In the normally developing adult the EMG should be silent when the person is relaxed and the muscle is passively stretched. Muscle tone in the adult is, therefore, mainly dependent upon biomechanical and not neurogenic mechanisms. The neonate on the other hand has active muscle tone which maintains her/his flexed adducted antigravity posture.

MEASUREMENT OF MUSCLE TONE
The resistance to movement which we call muscle tone can be measured in several ways: (1) upon perceived graded resistence to stretch which can be equated with the Ashworth scale; (2) an abnormal posture may be imposed on the limb e.g. decerebrate, hemiplegic, decorticate; (3) antigravity posture may be used as in pull to sit or the posture adopted in supine, prone and vertical suspended positions; (4) the range of joint motion is measured by goniometry which can be either simple manual or electronic. The range of movement is lessened in spasticity and increased in hypotonia.

MEASUREMENTS OF TONE USING TORQUE GENERATORS
The apparatus used (Fig. 9.14) has been described elsewhere (Lakie et al. 1984, 1988; Walsh 1992) A printed motor is a device eminently suitable for these observations as it can instantly convert a controllable electric current into the corresponding force. The motor has a double-ended shaft. One end is furnished with a light alloy handle of adjustable length and the joint is concentric with the motor; the fingers are held with a Velcro strap. The other end communicates via a metal boss with a low-friction conductive plastic potentiometer to record displacement.

133

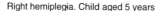

Right hemiplegia. Child aged 5 years

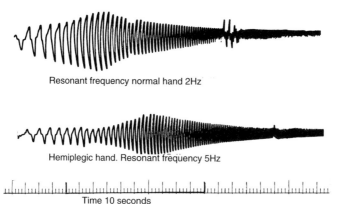

Resonant frequency normal hand 2Hz

Hemiplegic hand. Resonant frequency 5Hz

Time 10 seconds

Fig. 9.15. Higher resonant frequency in the stiff forearm muscles in a child with congenital hemiplegia.

As the frequency of the torque rises the oscillations increase to a maximum, the resonant frequency. With further increase the motion falls off. The resonant frequency varies with the state of the muscles being higher when there is voluntary stiffening. This measurement is useful for monitoring pathological conditions which give rise to hypertonia (Fig. 9.15). The wrist and associated anatomical structures behave as a torsion pendulum; the square of the resonant frequency reflects stiffness – a relation described in mechanical engineering textbooks (Walsh and Wright 1987). The equation is:

resonant frequency $= \frac{1}{2}\pi \sqrt{}$ (stiffness/inertia)

Thirteen children with hemiplegia aged 5 to 15 were tested. Some investigations were repeated over a period of 5 years (Brown et al. 1987). None of the patients were in the acute phase; all were on a clinical plateau. The resonant frequencies of the spastic hemiplegic limbs were significantly elevated (Fig. 9.16). The resonant frequency on the hemiplegic sides was 4.9 ± 2.3 Hz (mean and SD), and that on the normal side 2.3 ± 0.4 Hz. As the ages of the children varied, different levels of torque were used for different patients but for any one individual the torque values used were the same on the two sides.

With hypertonicity it is necessary to consider not only stiffness, as in a spring, but also damping, another cause of resistance to motion, as when trying to make any movement through treacle or heavy oil. Damping was investigated by dividing the velocity at resonance on the normal side with that on the hemiplegic side at the same peak torque level. The damping increased with increasing resonant frequency. perhaps due to the phasic stretch reflexes providing negative velocity feedback. This method of measuring muscle tone has been used by Corry and colleagues (1997) to follow the effect of botulinum toxin (type A) injection into the forearm muscles in children with congenital hemiplegia (see below).

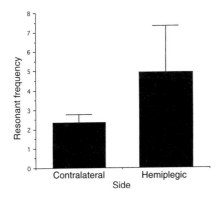

Fig. 9.16. Comparison of mean and standard deviation of the resonant frequency between the unaffected and the hemiplegic arm in 13 children with congenital hemiplegia.

SPASTICITY

Sherrington (1947) defined spasticity as implying increasing contraction and so resistance if stretch is applied to a muscle. In the experimental situation it can be defined as a stretch-dependent hypertonus which is abolished by posterior root section. There is no imposed resting posture since there is electrical silence at rest when there is no stretch. Rigidity on the other hand implies muscle contraction with EMG activity which does not require stretch to be applied to the muscle, is not abolished by posterior root section, but is driven from non-stretch receptors such as labyrinths, contact reactions and neck receptors.

BRISK REFLEXES AND PHASIC SPASTICITY

The most commonly accepted definition of spasticity is that of Lance (1981): "...a velocity-dependent increase in stretch reflexes and increased tendon jerks." There is, therefore, a simple short-duration, synchronous reponse to a sudden stretch. Rapid sinusoidal flexion and extension at a joint causes the classical clasp knife, i.e. a sudden contraction which rapidly melts away. We all have tendon reflexes but the velocity of stretch required to elicit them is normally outwith that used in everyday movements such as walking quickly, running, fast finger tapping or piano playing. If the threshold for eliciting the response is lowered then, apart from the clinical observation of brisk tendon jerks, the reflex muscle contraction may occur at normal speeds of movement so the patient complains that he cannot make rapid movements or s/he feels stiff, freezes and rapidly fatigues.

The velocity threshold, in the normally developing child, is usually greater than 50 degrees per second and may be over 200. The velocity of stretch imparted by a tendon hammer is much higher and may approach 400 degrees per second. If the speed of stretch is less than 15 degrees per second it does not excite the velocity-dependent annulospiral endings, even in the child with severe spasticity. Very slow flexion and extension of the limb, therefore, excites no resistance (Beradelli et al. 1982).

A phasically spastic muscle affects function as described above but shows a normal lengthening reaction, i.e. a normal extensibility which does not develop contractures and grows normally and does not appear to show secondary plastic biomechanical change.

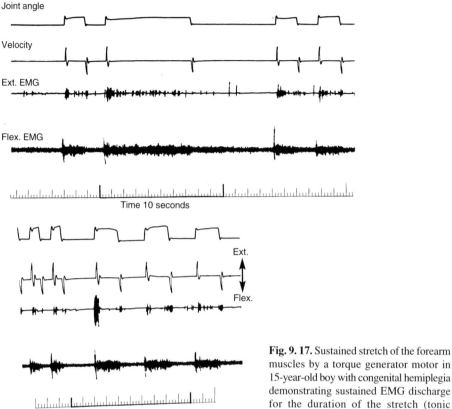

Joint angle

Velocity

Ext. EMG

Flex. EMG

Time 10 seconds

Ext.

Flex.

Time 10 seconds

Fig. 9. 17. Sustained stretch of the forearm muscles by a torque generator motor in 15-year-old boy with congenital hemiplegia demonstrating sustained EMG discharge for the duration of the stretch (tonic spasticity).

TONIC SPASTICITY

A tonic reflex is one in which the motor neurones produce a sustained asynchronous discharge which causes continuous recruitment and switching on and off of motor units producing a sustained smooth contraction of the muscle as a whole. In tonic spasticity as soon as the muscle is stretched it develops a reflex contraction, as shown by continuous EMG activity, independent of how fast it is stretched but lasting as long as it is stretched. This is what we mean by tonic spasticity. At rest, i.e. with no stretch applied, the muscle is electrically silent. Tonic spasticity tends to be maximum in flexors such as biceps, long finger flexors, pronators, and thumb adductors in the upper limb.

In our studies in Edinburgh, Scotland of upper- and lower-limb tone in children with hemiplegia such sustained responses were easily demonstrated using the torque generator motor and electromyography described above (Lakie et al. 1984). We found that the stiff forearm muscles showed a high resonant frequency, the EMG activity confirmed a short synchronous phasic response on rapid stretch followed on sustained slow stretch for the duration of the stretch i.e. tonic spasticity (Fig. 9.17) (Brown et al. 1987).

136

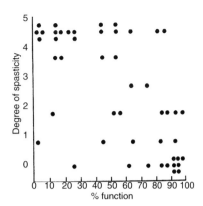

Fig. 9.18. Function plotted against the degree of spasticity in 49 children with congenital hemiplegia. A child may have no spasticity and no function or severe spasticity with preservation of function.

The secondary, flower-spray endings in the muscle spindle monitor sustained stretch. The secondary endings send their afferent impulses via the medial division of the posterior roots, having their cell bodies in the dorsal root ganglion. Although there is some monosynaptic connection most of the impulses are carried via second-order neurones, after synapsing in Clarke's column, in the dorsal spinocerebellar tract to the cerebellum.

The aim of rhizotomy is to remove the spindle input to the dorsal spinocerebellar tract. Spinal dorsolateral tractotomy, dentatotomy, cerebellar ablation and cerebellar stimulation probably act in the same way.

There is a statistical association of function with spasticity ($r = 0.74$ for clinical assessment and $r = 0.52$ for resonant frequency). In clinical practice function does not need to follow spasticity and in the individual case there may be no function and no spasticity or good function and marked spasticity (Fig. 9.18).

Tonically spastic muscle tries to stay at its shortest length, resists stretch even when applied very slowly, and shows reduced extensibility, i.e. the total lengthening reaction is less than the normal 1.8 times resting level. Spastic muscle is associated with reciprocal inhibition of its antagonist and so is not stretched normally when the antagonist contracts. The experimental demonstration by Tardieu of failure to add on sarcomeres if a muscle was not stretched for several hours a day added short-muscle disease as a major cause of fixed deformity in CP (Tabary et al. 1972). Tonically spastic muscle thus shortens and so develops a fixed contracture with even less lengthening. This is seen in the eventual fixation of the wrist drop, short finger flexors, short thumb adductor and secondary joint dislocations.

We thought that the interrelation of spasticity, deformity and contracture was finally settled by the concept of short muscles. Unfortunately biomechanical plastic change also appears to occur in these same muscles (Foley 1961). It is for this reason that one is often confused as to whether the stiff muscle is spastic, rigid, short or plastic. This probably explains why rhizotomy, baclofen, serial casting and botulinum toxin appears to work in some cases and not in others. Rhizotomy will not help in a rigid dystonic muscle but baclofen does, we do not know if botulinum toxin affects plasticity in muscle. Surgery is

137

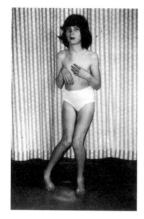

Fig. 9. 19. Posture of arm and leg in hemiplegia – arm internally rotated with wrist drop, leg internally rotated with foot drop. Unaffected side flexed to accommodate functionally shortened limbs on hemiplegic side due to fixed contractures, i.e. short muscles.

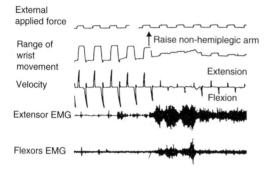

Fig. 9. 20. Gross increase in EMG activity and reduced range of movement produced by an externally applied torque on hemiplegic side as a result of using the unaffected limb.

best suited to short muscles and least to dynamic rigidity. The short-contracted long-finger flexors can be elongated by prolonged stretch as with serial casting.

Treating spasticity need not improve function, if the muscles are short there is a fixed flexion deformity at the wrist then the position is mechanically inefficient for movement. A better functional position can be obtained by a suitable thumb orthosis and is worth trying to see if a functionally better position improves the ability to use the poorly controlled digits (Currie and Mendiola 1987). A survey of 93 occupational therapists in the USA found no unanimity for or against splinting for spasticity (Neuhaus et. al. 1981). If one relieves spasticity by using botulinum toxin, for example, it does not cause an improvement in function. Surgical attempts to release the thumb and extend the wrist may produce a better cosmetic result but this rarely improves function as these abnormal postures are the result of spasticity and this does not directly relate to loss of skill which is proportional to loss of distal power and speed.

POSTURE OF THE LIMB

The upper limb in hemiplegia is usually maintained in a flexed posture at elbow, wrist and fingers and is internally rotated. The leg is extended at hip and knee with equinus at the ankle

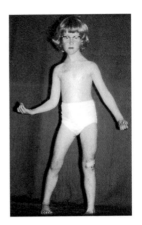

Fig. 9. 21. Externally rotated arm posture due to an increase in tone as an associated movement when trying to walk on outsides of feet (Fog test).

and is internally rotated – the hemiplegic or decorticate posture (Fig. 9.19). The flexed posture of the upper limb and extended lower limb is not due to spasticity but to uninhibited labyrinthine influences on basal ganglia free of cerebral cortical control. This can be demonstrated by turning the child upside down when the leg flexes and arm extends. The rotation at the shoulder also dictates the upper-limb posture, the arm most commonly being internally rotated, but in some children there is marked external rotation. The leg and arm tend to mirror one another; both being either internally or externally rotated – the former in congenital hemiplegia and the latter being more common in postnatally acquired hemiplegias.

The normal swing of the arm when walking is lost when the hemiplegic posture appears. Use of the unaffected hand causes a marked increase in tone in the affected side (Fig. 9.20) and this intensifies the hemiplegic posture. The effect of using the unaffected hand on the posture of the hemiplegic arm was marked in 10 of 24 children with hemiplegia in our own studies. The position of the lower limb also influences arm posture as shown in the Fog test – walking on the heels or with the feet inverted or everted heightens the hemiplegic posture (Fig. 9.21). Occasionally coughing, sneezing, yawning, laughing or stretching will result in sudden involuntary movement in a severely affected hemiplegic arm (Mulley 1982). Operations on the heel cord can thus aid the posture of the arm if this is being accentuated as an associated movement.

Some children have a more constant marked increase in tone which maintains an abnormal posture – a so-called dystonic hemiplegia. This can be predominantly flexor or extensor in the upper limb (Fig. 9.22), but is always extensor in the leg. Dystonic hemiplegias are more often associated with a deep white-matter infarct due to ischaemia in the territory of the lenticulostriate arteries. which affect the basal ganglia.

The abnormal tone is abolished by relaxation or shaking the limb when there may be a basal hypotonia. Dystonia must vary and is usually associated with cocontraction. Unlike spasticity it is not abolished by posterior-root section and so does not reduce after posterior rhizotomy. It is often GABA sensitive and may be reduced by benzodiazepines, baclofen or vigabatrin. Vibration, shaking or rhythmic action to music will also reduce dystonic rigidity.

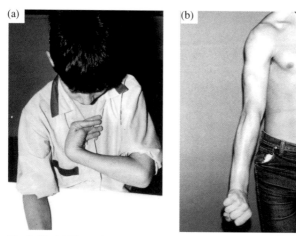

Fig. 9. 22. *(a)* Flexor dystonia in dystonic hemiplegia with hand in supination – Emu hand. *(b)* Extensor dystonic hemiplegia exaggerated by emotion and obstructed trying to walk through a doorway.

BIOMECHANICAL CHANGES IN MUSCLE

In a normal adult flexing and extending a joint allows the muscles to shorten or lengthen and this process is not accompanied by any electrical activity on the EMG and so is not associated with any electrically mediated muscle contraction. Any resistance, i.e. normal resting muscle tone, must be due to biomechanical and not electrically mediated resistance. The resonant frequency in these unaffected muscles will not change with surgical anaesthesia (Lakie et al. 1984). The range of movement at a joint, after tendon slack has been taken up, depends on the muscle paying out by allowing actin and myosin molecules to slide out of each other, thus elongating the sarcomeres. This is the extensibility of Tardieu. A muscle will normally lengthen by 1.8 times its resting length. The actual range of joint movement depends upon the total length of the muscle, i.e. the more sarcomeres, the more lengthening, and so the greater the range. Although it shows some elasticity, the tendon does not stretch sufficiently to allow movement without muscle elongation. If the muscle is stiff or sticky and actin does not slide through myosin (due to non neurogenic cross bridging, for example) there is increased resistance to movement, a decreased joint range and decreased extensibility.

PLASTICITY

If the child is examined rapidly in the clinic s/he may feel generally stiff with what appears to be spasticity with a fixed deformity. If a little time is spent and sustained pressure held for 10 to 15 seconds the resistance suddenly appears to melt away and a far greater range of movement at the joint becomes possible. In 1961 Foley demonstrated that the hypertonus at rest in adults and children with spasticity was independent of EMG activity. He showed very clearly the phenomenon of 'stress relaxation'. He also showed that physical therapy involving limb and trunk stretching could significantly reduce this type of muscle tone whereas complete peripheral nerve blocks had no effect.

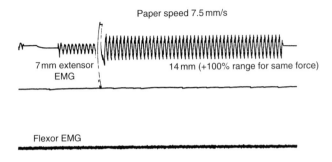

Paper speed 7.5 mm/s

7 mm extensor
EMG

14 mm (+100% range for same force)

Flexor EMG

Fig. 9. 23. Loosening following a brief disturbance. A thixotropic effect.

The plastic change appears to be a secondary phenomenon to the chronic neurological abnormality. It is thought that plastic change is the most important component of the peripheral biomechanical transformation which occurs in long-standing tonic spasticity. It offers a possible explanation of how serial casting can change the angle of a joint without changing power, length or degree of spasticity. It is why a child can be accommodated to an orthosis after repeated stretches and gives a scientific explanation of how physiotherapy can temporarily improve the child's activity and reduce tone. We still do not know if rhizotomy, baclofen or botulinum toxin will reduce plasticity (Foley's work described above suggests they will not) or if muscle relaxants such as sodium dantroline which mop up calcium would relieve the plastic resistance.

THIXOTROPY
'Thixotropy' is a plastic property of muscle which describes the effects of recent motion on muscle stiffness (Lakie et al. 1984). Limbering up loosens muscles; their stiffness depending on the previous history of movement (Fig. 9.23). This has been likened to a sol-gel conversion – as in shaking a bottle of tomato ketchup which is sticky when resting and more liquid after movement – which is attributed to the breakdown of weak physicochemical bonds which re-form when movement ceases. Thixotropic stiffness is independent of nerve supply and is not altered by muscle relaxants. Thixotropic stiffness is increased with cooling and movement is then ineffective in causing loosening. Thixotropy gives credence to the physiotherapy observation that putting joints through a full range of passive movements at the commencement of a therapy session increases the possible range of movements.

GROWTH DISTURBANCE
Growth disturbance is common and is more obvious in the leg as shortening than in the arm (Fig. 9.24) although comparison of finger nails will more easily demonstrate smaller fingers on the affected side. In 48% of hemiplegias dwarfing is present in the lower limb and the short leg imposes secondary changes such as pelvic tilt or a compensatory forefoot

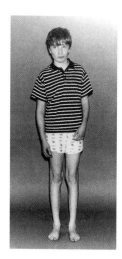

Fig. 9. 24. Short upper limb and smaller hand on hemiplegic side.

equinus. The bone age may be retarded in the hemiplegic compared to the unaffected side (Fig. 9.25). The bone mineral content was found to be reduced by 25% in the hemiplegic upper limb, lean muscle mass by 15%, but bone mineral density was well preserved as was the fat content (Lin and Henderson 1996). The more severe the functional impairment the worse the results – 22% reduction in lean muscle mass, for example .

VASOMOTOR CHANGES

Vasomotor changes occur in 25% of cases and show as a cold blue leg and foot with poor capillary return and chilblains in winter. Using the back of the hand as a sensor the foot is commonly found to be colder on the affected side. Conversely in an acute hemiplegia the leg may be warmer, pinker and swollen. It is said that in the cold, chronic erythrocyanotic limb there is increased vasodilatation in response to a different limb being placed in warm water. The skin is thin, shiny, heals poorly and the nails may be thickened and shrunken. It is not known whether these are autonomic effects with sympathetic excess due to loss of pyramidal inhibition. The autonomic nervous system is essential to increase the blood flow to a muscle during exercise. If this is blocked, as in beta blockade, marked muscle weakness results.

SENSORY DEFECTS

Sensory defects such as impaired pain, temperature, position and vibration sense are rare in congenital hemiplegia. Loss of two-point discrimination, texture sense, dysgraphaesthesia (recognition of shapes traced on the hand), astereognosis and finger agnosia are more common. Such sensory defects occur in about 28% of cases but the incidence depends upon the age at which testing is performed. Forty-five percent of normally developing children of 6 to 8 years with normal hand manipulation skills cannot tell shapes traced on her/his hand (dysgraphaesthesia), 30% have finger agnosia, 13% have mirror dyspraxia and 25% cannot obey commands for movements which cross the midline (Minns et al. 1977). Such recognition

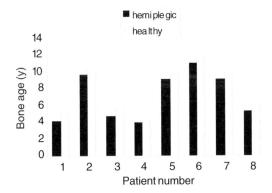

Fig. 9. 25. Comparison of bone age between normal and hemiplegic hand.

is developmentally determined so that to examine a child with hemiplegia at 8 years and say s/he has a sensory defect is meaningless. Disturbed two-point discrimination may be found on the normal upper limb in children with hemiplegia (Lesny 1971). Tactile extinction is significantly abnormal in the hemiplegic arm but again in a small number of cases may be ipsilateral to the side of the brain damage, particularly with a right hemiplegia (Lenti et al. 1991).

There may be delay in maturation on the affected side but there may be a more marked sensory loss on the unaffected side so the motor problem cannot be blamed solely on the sensory loss. If body image is tested throughout childhood the number of hemiplegic indviduals with difficulty gets progressively less. Rejection of a limb is not necessarily due to sensory loss and poor body image, but occurs also in association with severe dyspraxia. The output from muscle spindles and tendon organs responsible for spasticity do not reach consciousness and so when proprioception is tested it is not testing the motor sensory systems.

TREATMENT PROGRAM

We have explained the neurological basis for the wide variation in the components of a hemiplegia which account for the variation from child to child. Each component is amenable to a therapeutic program, as shown below, which needs to be tailored to the needs of the individual child. These have also been briefly described in the relevant section and are considered in detail elsewhere in the book. Unfortunately the paresis, i.e. degree of distal weakness, reflects the degree of brain damage and corticospinal dysfunction and the associated loss of function. Most of the therapies to the upper limb may objectively lessen muscle tone or improve the functional angle or cosmetic appearance of the limb but few have had proper clinical trials to show that function is improved. Treatment to the lower limb in order to improve gait and deformity has been better studied.

Distal weakness

An attempt to overcome the weakness can be made by an exercise program with a vigorometer or torque motor for example. It used to be a worry expressed by physiotherapists that exercise increased spasticity, but there is no evidence for this. If one calculates the quantity of EMG activity when eliciting spasticity and compares this to the amount of electrical activity on voluntary contraction it is seen that only a small portion of the muscle is involved in spasticity. Exercise of spastic muscle shows that power can be significantly increased. Therapeutic electrical stimulation can be applied at night while the child is sleeping. Creatine or anabolic steroids used to increase muscle bulk in atheletes have not been tried in children with CP but are sometimes tried in primary muscle disease. Biofeedback using EMG is used to try and give some sensory feedback in developing finely graded control of a finger movement. In severe cases some grasp can be restored by tendon transfer of brachioradialis to the extensor tendons of the finger (Pinzur et al. 1988).

Loss of skills

The practice of simple skills such as playing computer games or target practice and judgment-of-speed practice has been attempted. Equipment such as locating toy trains coming in and out of a tunnel has been specially designed for this. As one would expect, this is the area of greatest difficulty due to the 'cerebral' nature of the palsy and is the least likely to improve. Isolated voluntary movements, pathological associated movements and function were not found to be improved by careful EMG feedback training or conventional physiotherapy (Prevo et al. 1982).

Loss of speed

Speed is the last component of a skill to develop and depends upon frequent practice, it improves with age and also needs a warm limb.

Spasticity

Baclofen given orally is claimed to increase the use of the upper limbs (Minford et al. 1980). Botulinum toxin injected into the muscle will certainly reduce muscle tone (Fig. 9.26) but does not necessarily improve function (Corry et al. 1997). It may cause significant weakness but is a useful tool in assessing if temporarily relief of spasticity improves function or merely the cosmetic appearance. Introducing alcohol into the muscle is another method of temporarily relieving spasticity. Selective posterior rhizotomy is more often indicated in children with diplegia for relief of proximal spasticity in the legs rather than the upper limb in hemiplegia. In children with hemiplegia and severe seizure disorders who underwent surgical resection of the infarcted area of hemisphere it is claimed muscle tone significantly decreased and hand function improved (Di Rocco et al. 1993).

Velocity-dependent spasticity

This can be avoided by not rushing a task and slowing down the speed of attempted movement.

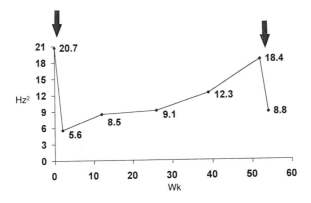

Fig. 9. 26. Graph of serial measurements of resonant frequency in a 14-year-old boy with a hemiplegia showing a sudden and marked drop in tone in the forearm muscles following the injection of botulinum toxin. (Corry et al. 1997).

Plastic change in muscle
Physiotherapy will temporarily relieve biomechanical change by putting the limb through a full range of passive movements, the limb should be kept warm and there is a place for 'warming up' before a therapy session. If wrist drop or deformity is due to plasticity in the muscles then a better position can be held by orthoses such as a 'cock up splint' after a period of stretching and exercising the muscle.

Failure of muscle growth
Failure of muscle growth, causes severe limitation in joint range and so may interfere with what voluntary function is present due to poor position such as a tightly flexed elbow, wrist drop of dislocated thumb. Stretching for several hours, at least 6 per day, is thought to be necessary in order to achieve sarcomere growth and so lengthening of the muscle. The stretch must be applied to a relaxed and not a competitively contracting muscle. This can be achieved by night splints or serial casting. Botulinus injection into the muscle may be necessary prior to stretch to relax the muscle. A combination of therapeutic electrical stimulation and splinting is claimed to be an effective combination (Carmick 1997). Surgery is necessary if the muscles are too short and do not respond to a stretching program. Tendon transfer and muscle release is claimed to improve grasp, grip strength and dexterity due to a better functional position of the wrist (Eliasson et al. 1998).

Abnormal postures
Vibration with a local vibrator applied to the muscle or use of a vibrating pad on which the child lies or rhythmic movement to music will all lessen dytonic posturing as will relaxation exercises. However, the effect is very transient. Do not try and splint or plaster a limb which is being held in an abnormal posture by dystonic muscle spasm or there is a risk not only of pressure sores but of ischaemic peripheral nerve damage. Lycra splints and suits

are less likely to cause interference with limb blood supply. In young children dystonic postures can be relieved by a benzodiazepine such as nitrazepam without making the child drowsy. A trial of possible efficacy can be made by giving intravenous diazepam after which the dystonia will immediately melt away if benzodiazepine sensitive. Baclofen given intrathecally by implanted pump will lessen dystonic rigidity and relieve pain in subluxed joints. A trial injection of Baclofen by lumbar puncture will show if there is likely to be any benefit. Surgical thalamotomy comes and goes in fashion as a treatment for dystonias, as there is a risk that speech may be made worse.

Sensory loss
An early stimulation program to try and establish body image and schemas for object weights, textures and so on should be part of an early intervention program. Stroking the limb, playing tactile rhyming games such as 'Round and round the garden' (an English rhyme which involves stroking the palm of the hand with a finger tip) are done instinctively by parents. Some physiotherapy programs include icing and brushing the stiff limb. Exploration by the good hand followed by the paretic hand in order to reinforce sensations of weight, texture, shape and temperature has been discussed.

Vasomotor changes
All that is usually needed to deal with this are warm gloves in winter to prevent frostbite. The importance of a warm limb to improve function is discussed above. The use of pharmacological agents such as nicotinic acid has the disadvantage that the rest of the body vasodilates so the child may be bright red everywhere but in the hemiplegic arm.

Retardation of bone age
A short limb is rarely an indication for surgery in the upper limb but quite frequently in the lower limb there is a need for shoe raises and more often nowadays limb-lengthening operations such as epiphyseal stapling.

Conclusion
A hemiplegia consists of several components which are independent of one another, such as loss of skills, distal weakness, loss of speed, brisk reflexes, velocity-dependent spasticity, length-dependent spasticity, plastic change in muscle, failure of muscle growth, abnormal postures, sensory loss, vasomotor changes and retardation of bone age. This is set against a variable horizon of cognitive ability, epilepsy, behavioural abnormality and so it is not surprising that no two children with hemiplegia appear to be exactly the same and there can be no universal prescription for treatment.

REFERENCES

Bell, Sir Charles (1833) *The Hand. Its Mechanism and Vital Endowments as Evincing Design.* London: Pickering.
Beradelli, A., Hallett, M., Kaufmann, C., Fine, E., Berenberg, W., Simon, S.R. (1982) Stretch reflexes of triceps surae in man. *Journal of Neurology, Neurosurgery and Psychiatry,* **45,** 513–525.

Bouza, H., Dubowitz, L.M., Rutherford, M., Pencock, J.M. (1994) Prediction of outcome in children with congenital hemiplegia: a MRI study. *Neuropediatrics*, **25**, 60–66.

Brodal, P. (1992) *The Central Nervous System Structure and Function*. Oxford: Oxford University Press.

Brooks, V.B. (1986) *The Neural Basis of Motor Control*. Oxford: Oxford University Press.

Brown, J.K., Van Rensburgh, F., Walsh, G., Lakie, M., Wright, G.W. (1987) A neurological study of hand function of hemiplegic children. *Development Medicine and Child Neurology*, **29**, 287–304.

— Minns, R.A. (1989) Mechanism of deformity in children with cerebral palsy. *Seminars in Orthopaedics*, **4**, 236–255.

Carmick, J. (1997) Use of neuromuscular electrical stimulation and dorsal wrist splint to improve hand function of a child with spastic hemiparesis. *Physical Therapy*, **77**: 661–671.

Carr, L.I. (1996) Development and reorganization of descending motor pathways in children with hemiplegic cerebral palsy *Acta Paediatrica*, **Suppl. 416**, 53–57.

Catalan, M.J., Honda, M., Weeks, R.A. (1998) The functional neuroanatomy of simple and complex sequential finger movements: a PET study. *Brain*, **121**, 253–364.

Chiron, C., Jambaque, I.,et al. (1997) The right brain hemisphere is dominant in human infants. *Brain*, **120**, 1057–1605.

Chollet, F., Di Piero, V., Wise, R. J., Brooks, D. S., Dola, R.J., Frackowiak, R, S. (1991) The functional anatomy of motor recovery after strokes in humans: a study with PET. *Annals of Neurology*, **29**, 63–71.

Corry, I.S., Cosgrove, A.P., Walsh, E.G., McLean, D., Graham, HK. (1997) Botulinum toxin A in the hemiplegic upper limb: a double blind trial. *Developmental Medicine and Child Neurology* , **39**, 185–193.

Currie, D.M., Mendiola, A. (1987) Cortical thumb orthosis for children with spastic hemiplegic cerebral palsy. *Archives Physical Medicine Rehabilitation*, **68**, 214–216.

Denckla, M.B. (1973) Development of speed in repetitive and successive finger-movements in normal children. *Developmental Medicine and Child Neurology*, **15**, 635–645.

Denny-Brown, D. (1966) *The Cerebral Control of Movement. Sherrington Lectures 8*. Liverpool: Liverpool University Press.

Di Rocco, C., Caldarelli, M., Guzzetta, F, Torriola, G. (1993) Surgical indication in children with congenital hemiplegia. *Child Nervous System*, **9**, 72–80.

Eliasson, A.C., Gordon, A.M., Forssberg, H. (1991) Basic coordination of manipulative forces in children with cerebral palsy. *Developmental Medicine Child Neurology*, **29**, 287–304.

— Ekholm, C., Carlstedt, T. (1998) Hand function in children with cerebral palsy after upper limb tendon transfer and muscle release. *Developmental Medicine and Child Neurology*, **40**, 612–621.

Foley, J. (1961) The stiffness of spastic muscle. *Journal of Neurology, Neurosurgery and Psychiatry*, **24**, 125–131.

Forssberg, H. (1998) The neurophysiology of manual skill development. *In:* Connolly, K. (Ed.) *The Psychobiology of the Hand. Clinics in Developmental Medicine, no. 147*. London: Mac Keith Press. p. 97–122

Friden, J., Lieber, R.L. (1996) Muscle architecture basis for neuromuscular control of the forearm and hand *In:* Wing, A. M., Haggard, P., Flanagan, J. R. (Eds.) *Hand and Brain. The Neurophysiology and Psychology of Hand Movements*. London: Academic Press. p. 69–79.

Gordon, A.M., Duff, S.V. (1999) Fingertip forces during object manipulation in children with hemiplegic cerebral palsy: I anticipatory scaling. *Developmental Medicine and Child Neurology*, **41**, 166–175.

— Charles, J., Duff, S.V. (1999) Fingertip forces during object manipulation in children with hemiplegic cerebral palsy: II bilateral coordination. *Developmental Medicine and Child Neurology*, **41**, 176–185.

— Forssberg, H. (1997) The development of neural control mechanisms for grasping in children. *In:* Connolly, K., Forssberg, H. (Eds). *Neurophysiology and Neuropsychology of Motor Development. Clinics in Developmental Medicine, Nos 143 and 144*. London: Mac Keith Press. p. 214–231.

Harrison, A., Connelly, K. (1971) The conscious control of fine levels of neuromuscular firing in spastic and normal subjects. *Developmental Medicine and Child Neurology*, **13**, 762–771.

Kim, S–G., Ashe, J., Hendrich, K., Ellerman, J. N., Merklt, H., Uğurbil, K., Gorgopoulos, A.P. (1993) Funtional magnetic resonance imaging of motor cortex: Hemispheric asymmetry and handedness. *Science*, **26**, 615–617.

Lakie, M., Walsh E.G., Wright G.W. (1988) Assessment of human hemiplegic spasticity by a resonant frequency method. *Clinical Biomechanics*, **3**, 173–178.

— — — (1984) Resonance at the wrist demonstrated by the use of a torque motor: an instrumental analysis of muscle tone in man. *Journal of Physiology*, **353**, 265–285.

147

Lance, J.W., McLeod, J.G. (1981) *A Physiological Approach to Clinical Neurology*. London: Butterworth. p. 128–148.

Lawrence, W. (1866) *Lectures on Comparative Anatomy, Physiology, Zoology, and the Natural History of Man*. London: Bell. (Original edition - 1819).

Lenti, C., Radice, L., Cerioli, M., Musetti, L. (1991) Tactile Extinction in Childhood Hemiplegia. *Developmental Medicine and Child Neurology*, **33**, 789–794.

Lesny, I. (1971) Disturbance of two point discrimination sensitivity in different forms of cerebral palsy. *Developmental Medicine Child Neurology*, **13**, 330–334.

Lin, J-P., Henderson, R.C. (1996) Bone mineralisation in the affected extremities of children with spastic hemiparesis. *Developmental Medicine and Child Neurology*, **38**, 782–786.

— Brown, J.K., Walsh, E.G. (1996) The maturation of motor dexterity or why Johnny can't go any faster. *Developmental Medicine and Child Neurology*, **38**, 244–254.

Minford, A., Brown, J.K., Minns, R.A. (1980) The effects of Baclofen on the gait of hemiplegic children – assessed by means of polarised light goniometry. *Scottish Medical Journal, Baclofen Symposium*. 29–35.

Minns, R.A., Sobkowiak, C.A. (1977) Upper limb fuction in spina bifida. *Zeitschrift fur Kinderchirurgie*, **22**, 493–506.

Molteni, B., Oleari, G., Fedrizzi, E., Bracchi, M. (1987) Relation between CT patterns, clinical findings and etiological factors in children born at term, affected by congenital hemiparesis. *Neuropediatrics*, **18**, 75–80.

Morgan, A.E., Aldag, J.C.(1996) Early idenitification of cerebral palsy using a profile of abnormal motor patterns. *Paediatrics*, **98(4)**, 692–697.

Mountcastle, V.B. (1997) The columnar organization of the neocortex. *Brain*, **120**, 701–722.

Mulley, G. (1982) Associated reactions in the hemiplegic arm. *Scandinavian Journal of Rehabilitation Medicine*, **14**, 117–120.

Nass, R. (1985) Mirror movement asymmetries in congenital hemiparesis. *Neurology*, **35**, 1059–1062.

Neuhaus, B.E., Ascher, E.R., Coullon, B.A., Donohue, M.V., Einbond, A., Glover, J.M., Goldberg, S.R., Takai V.L. (1981) A survey of rationales for and against hand splinting in hemiplegia. *American Journal of Occupational Therapy*, **35**, 83–90.

O'Regan, M., Brown, J.K. (1998) Neurological disorders and abnormal hand function. *In:* Connolly, K. (Ed.) *The Psychobiology of the Hand. Clinics in Developmental Medicine, no. 147*. London: Mac Keith Press. p. 241–261.

Penfield, W., Rassmussen, T. (1950) *The Cerebral Cortex of Man*. New York: Macmillan.

Pinzur, M.S., Wehner, J., Kett, N., Trilla, M. (1988) Brachioradialis to finger extensor transfer to achieve hand opening in acquired spasticity. *Journal of Hand Surgery*, **13**, 549–552.

Poore, G.V. (1873) Writer's cramp: its pathology and treatment. *Practitioner*, **10**, 341–350.

Prevo, A.J., Visser, S.L., Vogelaar, T.W. (1982) The effects of EMG feedback on paretic muscles and abnormal co-contraction in the hemiplegic arm, compared with conventional physical therapy. *Scandinavian Journal of Rehabilitation Medicine*, **14**, 121–131.

Rao, S.M., Binder, J.R., Hammeke, T.A., Bandetti, P.A., Bobholz, J.A., Frost, J.A., Myklebust, B.M., Jacobson, R.D., Hyde, J.S. (1995) Somatotopic mapping of the human primary motor cortex with functional magnetic resonance imaging. *Neurology*, **45**, 919–924.

Roland, P.E., Skinhoj, E., Lassen, N.A., Larsen, B. (1980) Different cortical areas in man in organisation of voluntary movements in extra personal space. *Journal of Neurophysiology*, **43**, 137–150.

Rothwell J. (1994) *Control of Human Voluntary Movement*. London: Chapman and Hall.

Rumeau, C., Tzourio, N., Murayama, N., Peretti-Vtion, P.,Levier, O., Joliot, M. (1994) Location of hand function in the sensorimotor cortex: M.R. and functional correlation. *American Journal of Neuroradiology*, **15**, 567–572.

Sherrington, C. (1947) *The Integrative Action of the Nervous System*. New Haven, CT: Yale University.

Spaulding, S.J., McPherson, J.J., Strachota, E., Kuphal, M., Raponi, M. (1988) Jebsen Hand Function Test : performance of the uninvolved hand in hemiplegia and of right handed, right and left hemiplegic persons. *Archives of Physical Medicine and Rehabilitation*, **69**, 419–422.

Steinlin, M.U., Good, M., Martin, E., Banziger, O., Largo, R.H. (1993) Congenital hemiplegia; morphology of cerebral lesions and pathogenetic aspects of MRI. *Neuropediatrics*, **14**, 224–229.

Tabary, J.C., Tabary, C., Tardieu, C., Tardieu, G., Goldspink, G. (1972) Physiological and structural changes in cat's soleus due to immobilisation at different lengths in plaster casts. *Journal of Physiology (Lond)*, **224**, 231–244.

Thelen E., Corbetta D.,Kamm K.,Spencer J.P., Schneider K., Zernicke R.F. (1993) The transition to reaching: mapping intention and intrinsic dynamics. *Child Development*, **64**, 1058–1098.

Thelen, E., Ronnqvist, L. (1988) Preparation for grasping an object: a developmental study. *Journal of Experimental Psychology: Human Perception and Performance*, **14**, 610–621.

Towers S. (1940) Pyramidal lesions in the monkey. *Brain*, **63**, 36–90.

Walsh, E. G. (1992) *Muscles Masses and Motion. The Physiology of Normality, Hypotonicity, Spasticity and Rigidity. Clinics in Developmental Medicine, No. 125*. London: Mac Keith Press.

— (1997) Synchronization of human finger movements: delays and sex differences with isotonic 'antiphase' motion. *Experimental Physiology*, **82**, 559–565.

— Wright G.W. (1987) Inertia, resonant frequency, stiffness and kinetic energy of the human forearm. *Quarterly Journal of Experimental Physiology*, **72**, 161–170.

Walshe, F.M.R. (1965) The problem of origin of the pyramidal tracts. *In: Further Clinical Studies in Neurology*. Edinburgh: Livingstone. p. 96–114.

Yousry, T.A., Schmid, U.D., Alkadhi, H., Schmidt, D., Peraud, A., Buettner, A., Winkler, P. (1997) Localisation of the motor hand area to a knob on the precentral gyrus. A new landmark. *Brain*, **120**, 141–157.

10
EPILEPSY AND HEMIPLEGIA INCLUDING STURGE–WEBER SYNDROME

J Helen Cross, Sarah E Aylett, and Jean Aicardi

An 'epileptic seizure' is a transient clinical event, a change in behaviour or movement arising from an abnormality of cortical neuronal discharge (Aicardi 1994). Epilepsy itself is a condition defined as one where the individual is prone to recurrent epileptic seizures, which implies more than two seizures. There are few studies examining the topic of epilepsy associated with hemiplegia in detail but most of these quote incidence figures that include children with a history of only one seizure, rather than recurring seizures. Such a definition is important, therefore, in this group of children and probably accounts for the variability in figures as summarised in Table 10.1; a history of at least one seizure is present in around 30 to 40% of children with hemiplegia (Perlstein and Hood 1954, Goutières et al. 1972, Ito et al. 1981, Uvebrant 1988) whereas 'active' epilepsy, that is children on treatment with or without continuing seizures is probably less common occurring in around 20% (Uvebrant 1988).

The risk of developing epilepsy in association with congenital hemiplegia appears to diminish as the child gets older with epilepsy presenting during the first 4 years of life in the majority of children. Goutières and colleagues (1972) found 44% of a group of 185 children with hemiplegia to have epilepsy. Twenty-seven percent presented with their first seizure under 1 year of age and 68% before 4 years. Thereafter, 28% presented between 4 and 10 years and 4% after the age of 10 years.

Seizure semiology
The seizure types that may present in children with hemiplegia are variable. It is difficult from a literature review to accurately summarise data on the frequency of seizure type, but two studies where data on semiology are available are summarised in Table 10.2. It could be assumed that the majority of individuals with hemiplegia would experience focal motor seizures, but startle seizures (Chauvel et al. 1992, Manford et al. 1996), negative myoclonus presenting as atonic drop attacks, and myoclonic jerks (Guerrini et al. 1998, Caraballo et al. 1999) have all been reported to be seen in association with different hemipathology.

As with focal epilepsy in general, the semiology depends on the area from which the seizures arise and further detail can be obtained with use of stereoelectroencephalographic (SEEG) studies. Chauvel has reviewed invasive EEG studies of 50 individuals with somatomotor seizures of frontal lobe origin; 20 had what was described as an infantile hemiplegia (and therefore assumed congenital hemiplegia), and a further 16 a hemiparesis

TABLE 10.1.
Prevalence of epilepsy in congenital hemiplegia

Study	n	With epilepsy (n)	%
Perlstein and Hood (1954)	384	144	43
Goutières et al. (1972)	182	81	43.8
Ito et al. (1981)	41	22	45
Claeys et al. (1983)	37	17	46
Uvebrant (1988)	134	37	28 (active 19%)

TABLE 10.2.
Prevalence of seizure types in hemiplegia

Type	Goutières et al. (1972) (%)	Uvebrant (1988) (%)
Partial seizures	74	69
Generalised tonic–clonic	27	46
Drop attacks	?	17
Infantile spasms	2.5	?

(Chauvel et al. 1992). In the infantile group, clonic seizures were seen with involvement of the primary motor cortex whereas tonic posturing was associated with widespread discharges on EEG extending to the whole of the motor and premotor areas.

More recent literature has suggested that startle-provoked seizures are relatively common in the hemiplegic population. Although this seizure type is not listed within older reviews of individuals with hemiplegia, this particular neurological abnormality makes up a significant proportion of studies of individuals with startle epilepsy, ranging from 26 to 85% (Table 10.3) (Agluglia et al. 1984, Chauvel et al. 1992, Manford et al. 1996). It is difficult to determine the relation of aetiology to this particular seizure type but there is a suggestion it is associated with ischaemic or acquired rather than developmental pathology. Eleven of 20 individuals in the series of Chauvel's group had a perinatal aetiology (Chauvel et al. 1992), as did, in Manford and colleagues' series, four of five individuals with a hemiparesis, all of whom had porencephalic cysts of an assumed ischaemic origin on imaging (Manford et al. 1996).

Startle-provoked seizures can be defined as those that occur in response to a startle stimulus, whether auditory (natural, particularly if sudden and intense) or somatosensory (tactile or mechanical, most commonly stumbling) but rarely visual (Chauvel et al. 1992, Manford et al. 1996). They may demonstrate motor features of a normal startle reaction, but in the majority of individuals spontaneous motor seizures are also seen with similar symptomatology. Asymmetrical posturing is due to involvement of the hemiparetic side, which causes increased amplitude and duration of tonic signs. As with the primitive startle reaction seen in the newborn child, repetition of the effective stimulus leads to habituation. The startle seizure represents the sensory precipitation of a motor attack of cortical origin. SEEG studies using depth electrodes suggest an origin of such seizures within abnormal

151

TABLE 10.3.
Prevalence of hemiparesis in startle seizures

Study	n	%
Aguglia et al. (1984)	9/16	56
Chauvel et al. (1992)	17/20	85
Manford et al. (1996)	?	26

motor and premotor areas of the frontal lobe (Chauvel et al. 1992), demonstrating either an exaggerated paroxysmal evoked potential or low-voltage fast discharge. There is subsequently very rapid spread of discharges, usually bilaterally. The age of onset range for this seizure type is wide; in all they appear to coexist with spontaneous seizures and in the majority are preceded by the onset of spontaneous seizures (Chauvel et al. 1992). There is also a tendency for this seizure type to manifest for the first time late in childhood or even adult life (Manford et al. 1996).

Developmental pathology, more specifically unilateral polymicrogyria with resultant hemiplegia has been associated with atonic drop attacks, atypical absence seizures and myoclonus. Some have shown increased weakness in the affected limbs during periods of frequent atonic seizures, with improvement after seizure control suggesting that the epileptogenic area included the motor cortex (Caraballo et al. 1999). The term negative myoclonus has been adopted due to the demonstration of loss of muscle tone during periods of spike–wave discharge (Guerrini et al. 1998). Such attacks can be rapid in occurrence, or slower and stepwise. This syndrome appears to be age specific (onset 2 to 5 years) and responsive to anticonvulsant drugs.

The above account is of specific seizure types but the most serious effects are seen in the epileptic encephalopathies where there is loss of cognitive function and quite often the development of psychiatric disorders. These encephalopathies include intractable hemiepilepsy of early onset with developmental arrest, West syndrome and continuous status epilepticus of slow sleep (ESES). Children with electrical status epilepticus of slow sleep (ESES) associated with multilobar polymicrogyria have been reported to have good outcome with regard to resolution but it is difficult to determine the degree to which cognitive function had been affected before and after ESES. Learning difficulties were apparent in all but one child with ESES, polymicrogyria and associated hemiplegia in one series (Guerrini et al. 1998) and all children in another series (Caraballo et al. 1999). Any child with congenital hemiplegia who shows cognitive arrest or deterioration should be suspected of developing an epileptic encephalopathy and be investigated by EEG including a sleep recording. These conditions in the majority require intensive medical treatment which may include corticosteroids, ketogenic diet and early assessment for surgical treatment. However, ESES associated with unilateral polymicrogyria may respond well to medication and has a good long-term outcome with regard to resolution (Guerrini et al. 1998, Caraballo et al. 1999).

TABLE 10.4.
TABLE 10.4.
Changes seen on the EEG in congenital hemiplegia

Study	Normal	Slow/diffuse change	Epileptiform
	%	%	%
Goutières et al. (1972)	35	-	41
Ito et al. (1981)	24	41	53
Uvebrant (1988)	23	28	20
Sussova et al. (1990)	12	20	48

Electrophysiology

Studies where children with congenital hemiplegia have undergone EEG have demonstrated that the EEG is abnormal in a greater number of children than the number diagnosed as having epilepsy (Table 10.4). Only 12 to 35% of EEGs performed in these children have been found to be normal. Not all abnormalities seen are epileptiform – spikes/sharp waves are seen in 20 to 50% and slow/diffuse changes in 20 to 40% (Goutières et al. 1972, Ito et al. 1981, Uvebrant 1988, Sussova et al. 1990). Although EEG abnormalities are not predictive of the development of epilepsy, Uvebrant (1988) found abnormalities in all 34 children with epilepsy in a group of 116 children with congenital hemiplegia who had undergone an EEG. Only 4% of children without known epilepsy had 'epileptiform' activity on the EEG. In addition, such changes are not only seen ipsilateral to the side of the lesion. Uvebrant found bilateral abnormalities or abnormalities predominantly on the side contralateral to the lesion in 15% and 9% of the children with epilepsy. Contralateral abnormality may be more apparent particularly in some aetiolgies where paucity of activity over the ipsilateral side may be seen. In a further group of children with hemiplegia undergoing presurgical evaluation, 17 of 21 children with congenital hemiplegia had bilateral abnormalities on interictal EEG (Doring et al. 1999). Abnormalities seen included discharges, abnormal slow activity, runs of rhythmic activity and abnormal fast activity. Such contralateral abnormalities were not an indication of poor postoperative success with regard to seizure freedom following hemispherectomy; indeed some resolved postoperatively. Outcome was more closely related to the underlying pathology; only 7 of 15 patients with developmental abnormalities became seizure free after surgery as opposed to 4 of 6 with middle cerebral artery infarcts.

As already outlined above, children who have demonstrated cognitive decline may have developed ESES, which can only be diagnosed by recording during sleep, and may be associated – although not exclusively – with polymicrogyria (Guerrini et al. 1998, Caraballo et al. 1999). Guerrini and coworkers quote a frequency of 18% in their series (Guerrini et al. 1998). In their group, however, because the course of ESES appears to be stereotypical and independent of brain damage and its cause, varying in duration but always ceasing before adolescence, age-related factors are thought to play a role in its genesis. Guerrini and colleagues (1998) suggest this to be age-related secondary bilateral synchrony (SBS) occurring through the corpus callosum. They also suggest age-related enhanced inhibition may contribute to the shift observed among their patients with unilateral polymicrogyria from initial early disinhibitory ictal acitivity (characterised by focal EEG abnormalities and focal seizures) to subsequent hypersynchronous spike and wave discharges that predominate during ESES.

Treatment

The principles of management should be followed as with any child with epilepsy. This consists of careful assessment of the nature of the attacks and a decision about the need for antiepileptic drug treatment based on the severity of the seizure disorder. There should perhaps be particular vigilance in view of the danger of compounding coexisting problems of learning and behaviour with anticonvulsant medication. As the majority of seizures within this group will have focal onset, first line anticonvulsants of choice should be carbamazepine or lamotrigine. However, certain anticonvulsants would be seen to have particular use in certain seizure types.

Vigabatrin had emerged as a useful drug in children with focal epilepsy with underlying cerebral structural abnormality, particularly in startle seizures associated with hemiplegia, although its use was limited by aggravation of behaviour problems and occasionally non-convulsive status epilepticus or myoclonic drop attacks. More seriously, its use has recently been curtailed because of visual field restriction after prolonged use and has meant that it is now confined to use in individuals whose visual fields can clinically be monitored and in whom vigabatrin is the drug that specifically controls severe seizures (Eke et al. 1997, Krauss et al. 1998). It is specifically contraindicated in children who already have a hemianopic field defect. Benzodiazepines, however, may also have selective use in the treatment of startle seizures. Alguglia and coworkers treated 16 patients with clonazepam or clobazam; of three treated with clonazepam two remained seizure free although problems were experienced with drowsiness and ataxia. This proved to be less of a problem in the 13 treated with clobazam, where 46% remained controlled for a mean 23 months although 15% were resistant and 38% experienced tolerance (Aguglia et al. 1984).

Prognosis

Although a relatively high proportion of children with congenital hemiplegia experience one seizure in a lifetime, only a small number go on to develop overt epilepsy. Despite the majority appearing to respond well to anticonvulsant medication, around a quarter of these children remain refractory (Uvebrant 1988). There is an association between epilepsy and learning difficulties; this is seen in epidemiological studies as well as in neuropsychological studies, where early onset of seizures are related to poor later cognitive outcome (Vargha-Khadem et al. 1991, see chapter 13). Epidemiological studies have included early onset epilepsy and underlying neurological disorder as associated with poor long-term outcome with regard to seizure control (Lindsay et al. 1979, Emerson et al. 1981, Brorson and Wranne 1987). Other small studies suggest a good outcome with regard to controlling seizures with some specific aetiologies (Guerrini et al. 1998, Caraballo et al. 1999). Children with congenital hemiplegia and early onset epilepsy, however, are likely to require long-term medication and experience ongoing seizures. Early referral for assessment for surgery in an attempt to control the seizures is paramount.

Sturge–Weber syndrome

One of the best known causes of epilepsy in association with hemiplegia is Sturge–Weber syndrome. The mechanisms of this relationship are becoming better understood. Sturge–Weber syndrome (SWS) is characterised by a facial capillary haemangioma (port wine stain, PWS) involving the periorbital area, forehead or scalp; a venous angioma of the leptomeninges (usually unilateral); and, in a proportion of cases, a choroidal angioma. SWS is a sporadic condition which is thought to result from failure of regression of a vascular plexus around the cephalic portion of the neural tube between 6 to 9 weeks' gestation (Shields et al. 1993).

The leptomeningeal angioma involves the pia mater, most commonly in the occipitoparietal region. A bilateral pial angioma occurs in 15% of cases (Bebin and Gomez 1988). Individuals with the radiological features of SWS, but without a facial PWS are described, but are rare (Oakes 1992, Sujansky and Conradi 1993). Occipital calcifications have been observed in association with epilepsy and coeliac disease, particularly in those with folate deficiency. (Gobbi et al. 1992). However, the other characteristic features of SWS were not present in these cases, and the pathology was distinct (Gobbi et al. 1992, Bye et al. 1993). In SWS, several layers of dilated veins and venous aneurysms lie within the subarachnoid space. On microscopic examination, there is calcification both within the vessel walls and in the parenchyma (Alexander and Norman 1960). Microgyria has been reported in SWS, and it is postulated that this is secondary to chronic ischaemia occurring in the prenatal period (Simonati et al. 1994).

Conventional angiography has shown decreased numbers of superficial cortical veins with enlargement of the deep medullary veins. There is a lack of normal venous drainage toward the superior longitudinal sinus through the superficial cortical veins, with drainage via the deep veins instead. This is associated with stasis and slowing of the venous circulation (Probst 1980). Sagittal venous thrombosis in SWS has been described, presumed to be secondary to the venous stasis (Benedikt et al. 1993).

Epilepsy

Epilepsy is reported in approximately 80% of individuals with SWS (Sujansky and Conradi 1995). Castroviejo and colleagues (1993) reported seizures in 32 of 40 children with SWS in a retrospective series. These figures are, however, derived from selected groups, and may not be fully representative of all cases. There are no epidemiological data relating to the incidence of SWS in otherwise asymptomatic individuals with a PWS. A questionnaire-based study sent to members of the SWS support group in the USA found that that the onset of epilepsy was within the first 2 years of life in 86%, and by 5 years in 95% (Sujansky and Conradi 1995). Seizures often occur during a febrile episode in infants (Castroviejo et al. 1993) and an early mean age of seizure onset at 5 to 6 months was associated with intractability. In a further retrospective series of 23 children with SWS, Arzimanoglou and Aicardi (1992) found a mean age of epilepsy onset of 31 months. Multiple seizure types were described, although partial seizures were most frequent. Almost 50% of this series had experienced episodes of status epilepticus, which were followed by the development of a permanent hemiplegia in a quarter of the children. Seizures were resistant to treatment in 15 of the 23. Acute episodes of epileptic encephalopathy occur in SWS with neurological deficit often becoming more severe after further episodes.

Electrophysiology

The EEG changes seen in SWS are of voltage attenuation over the area of the angioma, with a marked asymmetry in unilateral cases (Sassower et al. 1994). These changes are apparent early on in infancy. Interictal spikes ipsilateral to the lesion are, however, rare, while spikes may readily be seen in the contralateral hemisphere, with ictal recordings showing spikes often only at the periphery of the lesion. In two of the cases reported by Aylett and colleagues (1999) in which ictal recordings were carried out, slow activity was observed over the predominantly affected hemisphere consistent with the underlying ischaemic nature of the lesion.

Neuroimaging

The CT scan in SWS shows cortical atrophy and cortical calcification (Fig. 10.1a). There is enlargement of the choroid plexus, which is commonly bilateral (Terdjman et al. 1990). Cortical atrophy may involve one or more lobes, or both hemispheres in cases with a bilateral angioma. Cortical calcification is most commonly seen in the atrophic area and often has a gyriform appearance. Progression of cortical and subcortical atrophy and of calcification is reported in children followed prospectively with CT and MRI (Castroviejo et al. 1993). In infancy, white matter images suggestive of advanced myelination are commonly seen in the hemisphere underlying the angioma (Jacoby et al. 1987). However, accentuated T_2 shortening in the absence of accentuated T_1 shortening is against these findings being related to accelerated myelination (Barkovich 2000). It is postulated that observed T_2 shortening may in fact be related to an increase in deoxyhaemoglobin, secondary to the abnormality of the venous circulation.

Although CT may be helpful in those cases where calcification has developed, results may prove inconclusive in those cases where changes are more subtle, particularly in infancy. MRI with gadolinium is the diagnostic investigation of choice, demonstrating enhancement of the pial angioma (Benedikt et al. 1993) (Fig. 10.1b).

Regional cerebral blood flow using SPECT in SWS shows evidence of hypoperfusion of the affected hemisphere in cortical and subcortical regions (Chiron et al. 1989). Hypoperfusion is observed even in those cases where the imaging changes are subtle. However, a recent study suggests relative hyperperfusion of the affected hemisphere during the first year of life, with hypoperfusion seen after this time in both patients with and without epilepsy (Pinton et al. 1997). In addition to an abnormality of cerebral perfusion, positron emission tomography (PET) studies in children have shown reduced cerebral glucose metabolism (CMRGlc) (Chugani et al. 1989). The area of reduced CMRGlc was found to be more extensive than the area of abnormality seen on CT imaging. In the same study by Chugani and colleagues, two infants with SWS showed a paradoxical increase in CMRGlc within the affected hemisphere. The reasons for this are unclear, but could indicate that there is an age-related progressive change in CMRGlc in SWS as there appears to be in regional cerebral blood flow (Pinton et al. 1997). Data from Maria and coworkers (1998) suggests that progressive hypoperfusion and reduction of CMRGlc are associated with neurological deterioration in SWS.

Enhanced CT within a few days of episodes of prolonged seizures, has demonstrated cortical enhancement, with resolution of these changes on follow up at least 2 weeks later

156

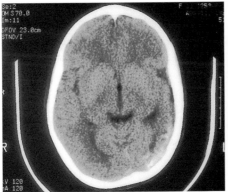

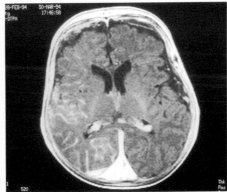

Fig. 10.1. CT scan calcification involving left parietal occipital lobes with associated left hemiatrophy

Fig. 10.2. Gadolinum enhanced axial MRI of infant aged 4 wk. This shows pial enhancement involving the right hemisphere. There is enlargement of the choroid plexus bilaterally.

(Terdjman et al. 1990). It is suggested that the transient enhancement is as result of a breakdown of the blood–brain barrier secondary to an impairment of vasomotor regulation during seizures. The suggestion that there is an insufficient increase in cerebral blood flow in response to seizures in SWS is supported by preliminary data from a study using transcranial Doppler to measure mean blood-flow velocity in the middle cerebral artery (MCA) (Aylett et al. 1999). In this study of three infants with SWS there was a reduction or lack of the expected increase in the MCA velocity of the predominantly affected hemisphere during clinical seizure activity. Riela and colleagues (1985) demonstrated evidence of an impairment of vasomotor reactivity to CO_2. These findings lend weight to the hypothesis that the vasomotor response to seizure activity may be insufficient in SWS. This could be a mechanism whereby seizures exacerbate the underlying ischaemic lesion (Chiron et al. 1987) and explain the seizure-related neurological deficits which are commonly observed.

With the further development of MRI techniques, quantitative diffusion has been used to assess a small group of infants and children with SWS (Kirkham et al. 1999). In two infants who had episodes of status epilepticus, there was a reduction in the apparent diffusion coefficient with hypointensity on T_2-weighted imaging. The three older children who had relatively well-controlled epilepsy did not show these changes. The reduction in the apparent diffusion coefficient and associated T_2 hypointensity could reflect the presence of compromised tissue associated with maximum oxygen extraction. Whether these findings are a reflection of the severity of encephalopathy in SWS, or an age-related phenomenon requires further prospective studies. Although there is evidence for an ischaemic mechanism operating in SWS, in theory, thrombosis within the angioma could also contribute to the observed acute neurological deficits. In addition, the authors are aware of two cases in which sagittal sinus thrombosis has occurred.

Outcome

Although transient or permanent hemiplegia frequently follows, and is exacerbated by seizures, focal weakness may be noted prior to the development of epilepsy (Sperner et al. 1990). Episodes of acute transient hemiplegia associated with migraine-like phenomena, but occurring in the absence of seizures appear to be common and are described in 30% of one series of children with SWS (Arzimanoglou and Aicardi 1992). There are theoretical reasons for suggesting the use of prophylactic low-dose aspirin in SWS to prevent the development of neurological deficit. There is some support for this from a review of children receiving regular aspirin who had a reduction in the frequency of acute episodes of hemiplegia (Maria et al. 1998). Further prospective data are needed to evaluate this. The combination of flunarizine, a calcium channel blocker, with low-dose aspirin may be helpful in those cases experiencing transient episodes of hemiplegia.

The cognitive outcome in children with SWS appears to be variable. In a retrospective series 12 of 40 children (mean age 9 years) were described as falling within the normal range, with 19 showing cognitive impairment which varied from mild (five children) to severe (eight children) (Castroviejo et al. 1993). Of those with the onset of seizures within the first year of life, 80% were reported as showing early developmental delay (Sujansky and Conradi 1995). Although a bihemispheric angioma appears to be associated with a poorer outcome (Bebin and Gomez 1988), it is noteworthy that in cases with unilateral leptomeningeal involvement, global cognitive impairment is common. Cognitive disability was found to be more common in those with an onset of epilepsy before 1 year and associated with a hemiplegia (Arzimanoglou and Aicardi 1992).

Barling and coworkers (1997) found that language skills were at a comparable level to cognitive ability in infants with SWS, but that there was evidence of fluctuation of both expressive and receptive language in association with seizure activity. Whether the abnormalities in language development are on the same basis as an epileptic aphasia or related to the underlying vascular abnormality requires further study.

Management

Surgical treatments for SWS have been used for over 40 years (Falconer and Rushworth 1960). The rationale behind their use has been the traditional epilepsy surgery model of removal or disconnection of the epileptogenic tissue, which in most cases requires hemispherectomy (Hoffman et al. 1979). Lobar resection can, however, be successful in appropriately selected children. Seizures often reduce in frequency (Ito et al. 1990), and the progressive cognitive decline may be halted or show some recovery (Vargha-Khadem et al. 1997). Acquired motor deficits in infants or children with an established hemiplegia following hemispherectomy are often minimal (Hoffman et al. 1979, Vargha-Khadem et al. 1997). The timing of such surgery appears to be crucial. Treatment very early in life, often before 1 year, appears to be more successful in abolishing seizures and ensuring more normal development (Hoffman et al. 1979). It is known from the use of hemispherectomy in other causes of intractable seizures as well as in SWS that early surgery is less likely to produce acquired motor, language or intellectual deficits. The difficulty with advocating early surgery for children with SWS, is that not all of them will show marked deterioration.

So a method of early prediction of those who will otherwise have a poor outcome is required in order to select those children who might benefit from early hemispherectomy. In those children where involvement is more localised, lobar excision may be associated with improvement in seizures, and may minimise postoperative deficit (Bye et al. 1989). In a recent series of 14 children who had been operated on, in seven where the angioma could be completely removed complete and lasting seizure control was obtained. In the remaining individuals, only one achieved complete seizure control (J Aicardi, A Arzimanoglou and F Andermann, personal communication).

Conclusion

Epilepsy is, therefore, a major factor in the clinical presentation, natural history, management and psychosocial outcome in about 20% of children with congenital hemiplegia. It is usually apparent early and may require intensive medical and sometimes surgical management.

REFERENCES

Aguglia, U., Tinuper, P., Gastaut, H. (1984) Startle induced epileptic seizures. *Epilepsia, 25,* 712–720.
Aicardi, J. (1994) *Epilepsy in Children, 2nd edn..* New York: Raven.
Alexander, G.L., Norman, R.M. (1960) *Sturge Weber Syndrome.* Bristol: John Wright and Sons. p. 57–68.
Arzimanoglou, A. Aicardi, J., (1992) The epilepsy of Sturge-Weber syndrome: clinical features and treatment in 23 patients. *Acta Neurologica Scandanavica (Suppl.),* **140,** 18–22.
Aylett, S.E., Neville, B.G.R., Cross, J.H., Boyd, S., Chong, K., Kirkham, F.J. (1999) Sturge-Weber syndrome: cerebral haemodynamics during seizure activity. *Developmental Medicine and Child Neurology,* **41,** 480–485.
Barkovich, A.J. (2000) *The Phakomatoses in Pediatric Neuroimaging. 3rd edn.* Philadephia, PA: Lippincott,Williams and Wilkins. p. 420.
Barling, E., Aylett, S.E., Sonksen, P., Stackhouse, J., Lees, J. (1997) Early speech and language development in Sturge-Weber syndrome – is it related to seizure activity? *European Journal of Paediatric Neurology,* **1,** A102.
Bebin, E.M., Gomez, M.R. (1988). Prognosis in Sturge-Weber disease: comparison of unihemispheric and bihemispheric involvement. *Journal of Child Neurology,* **3,** 181–185.
Benedikt, R.A., Brown, D.C., Walker, R., Ghaed, V.N., Mitchell, M., Geyer, C.A. (1993). Sturge-Weber syndrome:cranial MR imaging with Gd-DTPA. *American Journal of Neuroradiology,* **14,** 409–15.
Brorson, L.O., Wranne, L. (1987) Longterm prognosis in childhood epilepsy: survival and seizure prognosis. *Epilepsia,* **28,** 324–330.
Bye, A.M., Matheson, J.M., Mackenzie, R.A. (1989). Epilepsy surgery in Sturge-Weber syndrome. *Australian Paediatric Journal,* **25,** 103–105.
Bye, A.M.E., Andermann, F., Robitaille, Y., Oliver, M., Bohane, T., Andermann, E. (1993) Cortical vascular abnormalities in the syndrome of celiac disease, Epilepsy, bilateral occipital calcifications and folate deficiency. *Annals of Neurology,* **34,** 399–403.
Caraballo R., Cersosimo R., Fejerman N. (1999) A particular type of epilepsy in children with congenital hemiparesis associated with unilateral polymicrogyria. *Epilepsia,* **40,** 865–871.
Castroviejo, I.P., Diaz-Gonzalez, C.D., Garcia-Melian R.M., Gonzalez-Casado, I., Munoz-Hiraldo, E. (1993) Sturge Weber Syndrome: a study of 40 patients. *Pediatric Neurology,* **9,** 283–287.
Chauvel, P., Trottier, S., Vignal, J.P., Bancaud, J. (1992) Somatomotor seizures of frontal lobe origin. *Advances in Neurology,* **57,** 185–232.
Chiron, C., Raynaud, C., Nzourio, N., Dulac, O., Zilbovicius, M., Syrota, A.J. (1989) Regional cerebral blood flow by SPECT imaging in Sturge-Weber disease: an aid for diagnosis. *Journal of Neurology, Neurosurgery and Psychiatry,* **52,** 1402–1409.
Chugani, H.T., Mazziotta, J.C., Phelps, M.E. (1989) Sturge-Weber syndrome: a study of cerebral glucose utilization with positron emission tomography. *Journal of Pediatrics,* **114,** 244–253.
Claeys, V., Deonna, Th., Chrzanowski, R. (1983) Congenital hemiparesis: the spectrum of lesions. *Helvetica Paediatrica Acta,* **38,** 439–455.

Doring, S., Cross, H., Boyd, S., Harkness, W., Neville, B. (1999) The significance of bilateral EEG abnormalities before and after hemispherectomy in children with unilateral major hemisphere lesions. *Journal of Epilepsy,* **34,** 65–73.

Eke, T., Talbot, J.F., Lawden, M.C. (1997) Severe persistent visual field constriction associated with vigabatrin. *British Medical Journal,* **314,** 1693.

Emerson, R., DíSouza, B.J., Vining, E.P, Holden, K.R., Mellits, E.D., Freeman, J.M. (1981) Stopping medication in children with epilepsy: predictors of outcome. *New England Journal of Medicine,* **304,** 1125–1129.

Falconer, M.A., Rushworth, R.G. (1960) Treatment of encephalotrigeminal angiomatosis (Sturge-Weber disease) by hemispherectomy. *Archives of Disease in Childhood,* **35,** 433–447.

Gobbi, G., Bouquet, F., Greco, L., Lambertini, A., Tassinari, C.A., Ventura, A., Zaniboni, M.G. (1992) Coeliac disease, epilepsy, and cerebral calcifications. *Lancet,* **340,** 439–443.

Goutières, F., Challamel, M-J., Aicardi, J., Gilly, R. (1972) Les Hemiplegies Congenitales: Semiologie, eitiologie et pronostic. *Archives Francaises Pédiatriques,* **29,** 839–851.

Guerrini, R., Genton, P., Bureau, M., Parmeggiani, A., Sala-Puig, X., Santucci, M., Bonanni, P., Ambrosetto, G., Dravet, C. (1998) Multilobar polymicrogyria, intractable drop attack seizures, and sleep-related electrical status epilepticus. *Neurology,* **51,** 504–512.

Hoffmann, H.J., Hendrick, E.B., Dennis, M., Armstrong, D. (1979) Hemispherectomy for Sturge-Weber syndrome. *Child's Brain,* **5,** 233–248.

Ito, M., Okuno, T., Takao, T., Konishi, Y., Yoshioka, M., Mikawa, H. (1981) Electroencephalographic and cranial computed tomographic findings in children with hemiplegic cerebral palsy. *European Neurology,* **20,** 312–318.

— Sato, K., Ohnuki, A., Uto, A. (1990) Sturge-Weber disease: operative indications and surgical results. *Brain and Development,* **12,** 473–477.

Jacoby, C.G., Yuh, W.T.C., Afifi, A.K., Bell, W.E., Schelper, R.L., Sato, Y. (1987) Accelerated myelination in early Sturge-Weber syndrome demonstrated by MR imaging. *Journal of Computer Assisted Tomography,* **11,** 226–231.

Kirkham, F.J., Calamante, F., Bynevelt, M., Aylett, S., Porter, D.A., Chong, W.K, Gadian, D.G., Connelly, A (2000) Quantitative diffusion imaging studies in Sturge-Weber syndrome. *Developmental Medicine and Child Neurology,* **41, suppl. 82,** 16–17. (Abstract).

Krauss, G.L., Johnson, M.A., Miller, N.R. (1998) Vigabatrin-associated retinal cone dysfunction: electroretinogram and ophthalmologic findings. *Neurology,* **50,** 614–618.

Lindsay, J., Ounsted, C., Richards, P. (1979) Longterm outcome in children with temporal lobe seizures I: social outcome and childhood factors. *Developmental Medicine and Child Neurology,* **21,** 285–298.

Manford, M.R., Fish, D.R., Shorvon, S.D. (1996) Startle provoked epileptic seizures: features in 19 patients. *Journal of Neurology, Neurosurgery and Psychiatry,* **61,** 151–156.

Maria, B.L., Neufeld, J.A., Rosainz, L.C., Drane, W.E., Quisling, R.G., Ben-David, K., Hamed, L.M. (1998) Central nervous system structure and function in Sturge Weber Syndrome: evidence of neurologic and radiologica progression. *Journal of Child Neurology,* **13,** 606–618.

Oakes, W. J. (1992) The natural history of patients with Sturge-Weber syndrome *Paediatric Neurosurgery,* **18,** 287–290.

Perlstein, M. A., Hood, P. N. (1954) Infantile spastic hemiplegia I. Incidence. *Pediatrics,* **14,** 436–441.

Pinton, F., Chiron, C., Enjolras, O., Motte, J., Syrota, A., Dulac, O. (1997) Early single photon emission computed tomography in Sturge Weber syndrome. *Journal of Neurology, Neurosurgery, Psychiatry,* **63,** 616–621.

Probst, F.P. (1980) Vascular morphology and angiographic flow patterns in Sturge-Weber angiomatosis:facts, thoughts and suggestions. *Neuroradiology,* **20,** 73–78.

Riela, A., Stump, D., Roach, S. (1985) Regional cerebral blood flow characterisitics of the Sturge-Weber syndrome. *Pediatric Neurology,* **1,** 85–90.

Sassower, K., Duchowny, M., Jayakar, P., Resnick, T., Levin, B., Alvarez, L., Dean, P.J. (1994) EEG evaluation in children with Sturge-Weber syndrome and epilepsy. *Epilepsia,* **7,** 285–289.

Shields, W.D., Duchowny, M., Holmes, G. (1993) Surgically remediable syndromes of infancy and early childhood. *In:* Engel, J. Jr. (Ed) *Surgical Treatment of the Epilepsies, 2nd edn.* New York: Raven Press. p. 35–48.

Simonati, A., Colamaria, V., Bricolo, A., Dalla Bernardina, B., Rizzuto, N. (1994) Microgyria associated with Sturge-Weber angiomatosis *Child's Nervous System,* **10,** 392–395.

160

Sperner, J., Schmauser, I., Bittner, R., Henkes, H., Bassir, C., Sprung, C., Scheffner, D., Felix, R. (1990) MR-Imaging findings in children with Sturge-Weber syndrome. *Neuropediatrics,* **21,** 146–152.

Sujansky, E., Conradi, S. (1995) Outcome of Sturge-Weber syndrome in 52 adults. *American Journal of Medical Genetics,* **57,** 35–45.

Süssova, J., Seidl, Z., Faber J. (1990) Hemiparetic forms of cerebral palsy in relation to epilepsy and mental retardation. *Developmental Medicine and Child Neurology,* **32,** 792–795.

Terdjman, P., Aicardi, J., Sainte-Rose, C., Brunelle, F. (1990) Neuroradiological findings in Sturge-Weber syndrome (SWS) and isolated pial angiomatosis. *Neuropediatrics,* **22,** 115–120.

Uvebrant, P. (1988) Hemiplegic cerebral palsy aetiology and outcome. *Acta Paediatrica Scandinavica,* **s345,** 65–67.

Vargha-Khadem, F., Isaacs, E., van der Werf, S., Robb, S., Wilson,J. (1992) Development of intelligence and memory in children with hemiplegic cerebral palsy: The deleterious consequences of early seizures. *Brain,* **115,** 315–329.

— Carr, L., Isaacs, E., Brett, E., Adams, C., Mishkin, M. (1997). Onset of speech after left hemispherectomy in a nine year old boy. *Brain,* **120,** 159–182.

11
HEMISPHERECTOMY IN CONGENITAL HEMIPLEGIA

Brian Neville

Hemispherectomy has been used for the treatment of intractable hemiepilepsy in association with congenital hemiplegia for the past 60 years. It has been clear for most of this time that when there are totally concordant data lateralising seizure source and pathology this is the epilepsy surgery procedure with the highest rate of seizure relief. Interestingly, this, the most major of interventions, has not been discussed in the context of habilitation of the primary disabling condition of congenital hemiplegia. It is, however, important that those managing developmental impairments of both young and older children are clear about the indications for investigation and surgical treatment of epilepsy and are prepared to provide postoperative rehabilitation.

In principle there are two types of surgical operation for epilepsy: resection and disconnection procedures. Surgical resection for epilepsy relies upon the following evidence:

(1) The epilepsy arises from one part of the brain using evidence from the clinical seizure semiology, neurophysiology and other functional data, e.g. ictal single photon emission computed tomography (SPECT);

(2) There is ideally a single, neuroradiologically identifiable lesion concordant with the functional evidence of seizure source.

(3) The lesion and epileptogenic area of the brain are safely removable either because they are in the relatively non-eloquent cortex or because the functions carried out by that part of the brain have already been lost or relocated.

Although resection and disconnection procedures have been regarded as being different in principle, this distinction may be artificial in the context of hemispherectomy because the most commonly used procedures rely predominantly on disconnection. Also, although the stated primary aim of the procedure is to stop seizures by resection or disconnection, the second and equally important purpose is to prevent the discharging hemisphere from interfering with the development and functioning of the other hemisphere. Evidence for the adverse developmental effects of clinical and subclinical seizures is now overwhelming and is one of the key issues in selecting children for surgical treatment. From the early experience of hemispherectomy for epilepsy it became clear that there was a gratifying recovery from the severe behaviour problems that commonly coexist, in those whose epilepsy stopped. This is discussed further in chapter 12.

A number of techniques have been used under the term hemispherectomy and briefly the techniques available are as follows:

(1) Anatomical hemispherectomy. This operation as developed by Dandy (1928) for the treatment of tumours involved complete removal of the white and grey matter of the hemisphere with preservation of the thalamus although later modifications used for the treatment of epilepsy tended to preserve the basal ganglia. Despite it being apparent that this was a good operation for the relief of epilepsy and related behavioural problems there was an unacceptable complication rate of hydrocephalus and superficial cerebral haemosiderosis. This latter complication consisted of subpial iron deposition with inflammatory and gliotic changes causing a progressive neurological deterioration with an ultimately fatal outcome in 25% of patients (Oppenheimer and Griffith 1966). For this reason the procedure was abandoned temporarily and a range of modified procedures introduced to reduce the size of the hemispherectomy cavity.

(2) Modified hemispherectomy consists of an anatomical hemispherectomy, occlusion of the foramen of Munro with muscle and stripping of the dura from the skull vault fixing it to the falx, tentorium and middle fossa (Wilson 1970 and Adams 1983.)

(3) Hemidecortication. In this procedure the grey matter is stripped off the hemisphere leaving the white matter intact.

(4) Functional hemispherectomy consists of a large fronto-parieto-temporal resection with complete cortical disconnection of the remaining parts of the hemisphere and usually undermining the insula cortex.

(5) Hemispherotomy is the ultimate cavity-preventing procedure in which disconnection including callosotomy and undermining of the hemisphere through the ventricle is achieved from either a vertex (Delalande et al 1992) or lateral (Villemure 1997) approach.

All of the above procedures have the same functional aim of protecting the unaffected hemisphere from epileptic discharges and are probably of equal efficacy in experienced hands. However, if a functional procedure fails and the evidence indicates that the continuing seizures are arising from the supposedly disconnected hemisphere a modified anatomical hemispherectomy may be offered.

Hemispherectomy is a major procedure and complications may occur but superficial cerebral haemosiderosis has not been reported with any of the new procedures (Villemure 1997).

The pathologies causing intractable hemiepilepsy are nearly as wide as those causing congenital hemiplegia except that epilepsy is rare in periventricular leukomalacia. These pathologies are discussed in chapters 2 and 10. There is a clear difference in the predicted outcome of hemispherectomy depending on pathology. With a major migration defect of the hemisphere, for example, only about 60% of patients achieve freedom from seizures whereas with acquired intrauterine damage, such as middle cerebral infaction, between 80% and 90% achieve seizure freedom. The reasons for this are not clear, although one might suspect that with such a major, apparently unilateral, brain malformation of hemimegalencephaly that there may well be abnormality of the other hemisphere. There is very little evidence to support this notion. With hemimegalencephaly and very early (probably intrauterine) onset of seizures, development is severely delayed, and although current surgery allows development to proceed, cognitive function does not usually exceed an IQ of 50. An example of the management of a child with hemimegalencephaly illustrates these issues.

Case study

This boy presented with obvious seizures from 8 months of age. From the neonatal period jerks of the head to the left were observed and these developed into partial motor seizures of the left arm and leg with secondary generalisation occurring at a high rate from 8 months. There was an excessive rate of head growth and a typical scalp lesion of the linear sebaceous naevus syndrome. MRI scan at 11 months showed right hemimegalencephaly with a cystic lateral ventricle and a radiologically normal left hemisphere. He had a left hemiparesis and showed reaching and exploring with his right hand. No language development had occurred but he was alert and friendly. He had a dense left homonomous hemianopia. His development was at a 6-month level at 11 months and had reached a plateau. EEGs showed virtually continuous discharges over the right hemisphere. Sodium valproate and carbamazepine were ineffective but phenytoin and phenobarbitone produced control of all clinical seizures for 1 year but they recurred from age 2:1 years (2 years, 1 month). During this time an EEG showed continuing severe epileptic abnormality over the right hemisphere. His development had made only very slow progress with a peak at 19 months and then regression with overall development at a 15-month level at 2:5 years. He had a very short attention span. He could pull to stand but could not walk independently.

A right functional hemispherectomy was performed when the patient was aged 2:7 years. His seizures stopped. The hemiparesis was temporarily worse but he regained hand grasp and walked for the first time within 4 months of surgery.

Following this he made slow progress but with development at a rate of less than 50% that of a normally developing child. Seizures then returned and, therefore, an anatomical hemispherectomy was performed aged 4:2 years following which he was seizure free and was weaned off antiepileptic drugs. When reviewed at 4:10 years, he was lively and interactive in marked contrast to his obtunded state before the first operation. He was using speech appropriately and the surgery was regarded as successful.

He made steady motor progress despite the increased motor deficit. There were problems in getting an ankle–foot orthosis (AFO) that would correct the mobile valgus deformity.

This boy illustrates the need for early active enquiry into why a young child with congenital hemiplegia is falling behind developmentally. Epilepsy and particularly subclinical epilepsy must be suspected as being the cause of a substantial part of the developmental delay. Our starting position should be that there is no reason why a child with one unaffected hemisphere should not have abilities within the normal range unless there is some other factor interfering with learning. It is, therefore, helpful to have an early MRI scan to see if the lesion has a high chance of being epileptogenic as in the case above. Developmental arrest or regression in this context should be investigated up to and including a sleep EEG record. The severity of the hemiparesis may be difficult to assess at an early age when there is a high rate of seizures contributing to a variable but more-or-less continuous postictal weakness and disuse. A predictive judgement has to be made about the relative likelihood of there being significant use of the limb in the context of continuing seizures as against the cognitive, social and behavioural effects of continuing clinical seizures. Increasingly it is believed that early surgery should be considered in this context and that much of the damage has probably occurred in the first 6 months of life. We would now suggest earlier surgery for the child discussed above on the basis of developmental arrest and subclinical epileptic status.

Problems in managing the foot and ankle following early hemispherectomy are probably due to loss of postural feedback producing a strong tendency for the ankle to fall into valgus. Orthotists vary in their ability to produce AFOs that fit young children closely enough to correct such coronal-plane abnormalities and to do so without causing skin damage.

The reasons for recurrence of seizures in the case quoted seem likely to be residual connected epileptogenic foci within the malformed hemisphere. The first procedure had, however, produced dramatic developmental improvement. The tendency for a relatively poor cognitive and seizure-free outcome in major dysplastic lesions rather than with later intrauterine strokes emerges from many series (Holthausen et al. 1997). The cognitive penalty seems likely to be due to early and often intrauterine onset of seizures. The poorer seizure outcome in hemimegalencephaly seems likely to be multifactorial with greater technical difficulty with functional disconnections and the greater theoretical likelihood of contralateral lesions.

Conclusion

In summary, hemispherectomy is often an extremely successful intervention to halt disabling siezures (and accompanying behavioural problems and cognitive decline) that have not been controllable by other means. The main disadvantage is further deterioration in motor and sensory function on the affected side if there is not already a dense hemiplegia and hemianopia. Operative risks are low and late complications rare. The operation is underused and should actively be considered in children and adults with early onset of hemiplegia and seizures that continue despite the use of three antiepilepsy drugs. In young children with very severe hemiepilepsy there is a developing consensus on the need for urgent referral.

REFERENCES

Adams, C.B.T. (1983) Hemispherectomy: a modification. *Journal of Neurology, Neurosurgery and Psychiatry,* **46,** 617–619.
Dandy, W. (1928) Removal of right cerebral hemisphere for certain tumors with hemiplegia. *Journal of the American Medical Association,* **90,** 823–825.
Delalande, O., Pinard, J.M., Basdevant, C., Gauthe, M., Plouin, P., Dulac, O. (1992) Hemispherectomy: a new procedure for central disconnection. *Epilepsia,* **33(Suppl. 3),** 99–100.
Holthausen, H., May, T. W., Adams, C. T. B., et al. (1997) Seizures post hemisherectomy. *In:* Tuxhorn I, Holthausen H, Boenigk HE, (Eds.) *Paediatric Epilepsy Syndromes and Their Surgical Treatment.* London: John Libbey and Company, p. 749–773.
Oppenheimer, D.R. Griffith, H.B. (1966) Persistent intracranial bleeding as a complication of hemispherectomy. *Journal of Neurology, Neurosurgery and Psychiatry,* **9,** 229–240.
Wilson, P.J.E. (1970) Cerebral hemispherectomy for infantile hemiplegia. *Brain,* **93,** 147–180.
Villemure, J.G. (1997) Hemispherectomy techniques: a critical review. *In:* Tuxhorn I, Holthausen H, Boenigk HE, (Eds.) *Paediatric Epilepsy Syndromes and Their Surgical Treatment.* London: John Libbey and Company, p. 729–738.

12
EMOTIONAL, BEHAVIOURAL AND SOCIAL CONSEQUENCES

Robert Goodman and Carol Yude

Many professionals seem to think of childhood hemiplegia as amounting to no more than a mild physical disability. This is not how it generally seems to the children themselves or their families. First, what may look like a mild physical problem to a paediatrician or physiotherapist who is used to working with children with quadriplegia or muscular dystrophy often does not seem mild to the person involved. It is not a minor matter always to be last on sports day and never to be chosen for a school team. Nor is it a minor matter to need help cutting up your food, doing up your shoelaces, or to be unable to carry your tray in the school canteen. These sorts of things can make children uncomfortably conspicuous and thereby make school life more stressful and less rewarding. In addition, as described in this chapter and chapter 13, many children with hemiplegia have relatively 'invisible' psychological problems that make a major difference to the child's life. These can include specific learning difficulties, generalised learning difficulties, anxiety, depression, hyper-activity, behavioural difficulties, autistic problems and social isolation. The child's life is often more disrupted by the psychological difficulties associated with hemiplegia than by the hemiplegia itself. Consequently, all professionals who come into regular contact with children who have hemiplegia need to be psychologically minded so that psychological problems are recognised and appropriate help provided. Sometimes this help can come from 'front-line' professionals such as teachers, physiotherapists or community paediatricians. In other instances, referral to specialist mental-health professionals will be needed.

Early studies

Evidence that childhood hemiplegia is associated with an increased rate of emotional difficulty goes back some 50 years. Some of the earliest reports are about children with hemiplegia who had a hemispherectomy operation (see chapter 11). For example, in Krynauw's (1950) pioneering description of hemispherectomy for children with hemiplegia and intractable epilepsy, he emphasised severe behavioural and social problems and wrote that "in the cases that have come under my observation it has been the mental state that has impressed me most strongly, and in many, it has been the mental state, rather than the hemiplegia and epilepsy, which has led the parents to seek advice" (p. 243). In many cases, both in Krynauw's series and in subsequent series, the hemispherectomy operation not only abolished or improved seizures but reportedly led to a marked improvement in behaviour too.

Children who came to hemispherectomy were clearly not typical of children with congenital hemiplegia in general, but other early studies showed that behavioural problems were not simply confined to those children with intractable seizures. The two classical descriptions of the hyperkinetic syndrome – involving severe and pervasive hyperactivity and inattention – both demonstrated a link with childhood hemiplegia. Ounsted (1955) reported a high rate of hyperkinesis among children with epilepsy, particularly when the children also had hemiplegia: 31% of children with epilepsy and hemiplegia also showed the hyperkinetic syndrome, as compared with 7% of children with epilepsy but no hemiplegia. In Ingram's (1955) study of a representative sample of children with cerebral palsy (CP), he also noticed a high rate of hyperkinesis, affecting 12% of the children with hemiplegia as compared with 5% of children with other cerebral palsies. In a subsequent paper, Ingram (1956) provided more details on eight children with hemiplegia and hyperkinesis; it was particularly note-worthy that five of the eight children did not have seizures, and a similar proportion had a mild hemiparesis. The link between hemiplegia and hyperactivity clearly could not be attributed solely to the consequences of epilepsy or antiepileptic medication.

Early studies also made it clear that chronic neurodevelopmental problems were associated with a broad range of psychological problems and not just with hyperactivity. Ingram (1955) reported that the majority of his representative sample of children with CP showed behavioural disorders at some time or another. The conclusion that many children with CP have associated psychiatric problems also emerged from the subsequent neuropsychiatric study by Rutter, Graham and Yule (1970) on the Isle of Wight: psychiatric disorders were present in 44% of children with CP and an IQ of at least 50, as compared with 12% of children with chronic physical disorders not involving the cerebral hemispheres, and 7% of children with no physical disorders. This Isle of Wight study was a landmark in demonstrating that children with chronic neurodevelopmental disorders were at a substantially higher risk of developing psychiatric problems than were other children, even when these other children had chronic physical disorders. Subsequent studies have provided further evidence for direct brain–behaviour links over and above the psychological distress related to any form of chronic disability or illness (Seidel et al. 1975, Breslau 1985). The Isle of Wight study demonstrated that chronic neurodevelopmental disorders were associated with an increased rate of many different sorts of psychiatric problems, including emotional, hyperactivity and conduct disorders. There was no one 'brain-damage syndrome'. Since the Isle of Wight sample only included 11 children with congenital or acquired hemiplegia it was obviously not possible to examine how far these general conclusions applied to hemiplegia specifically.

Recent studies

Studies to estimate the frequency of psychological problems in hemiplegia need to be conducted on representative samples rather than clinic samples. This is to avoid selection bias which typically leads to children with complex and severe problems being overrepresented in clinics. In recent years, two large and representative samples of children with hemiplegia have been studied from a behavioural perspective. Uvebrant (1988) studied a representative sample of Swedish children with hemiplegia (also see chapter 5). Severe hyperkinetic behaviour and attention deficit were recorded in 6 of 111 (5.4%) children with congenital hemiplegia in the absence of learning disability. Though no control group was included, this is probably three to five times commoner than would be expected in a comparable sample of children without any physical disability.

The London Hemiplegia Register (LHR) study (Goodman and Graham 1996) has also used a large and representative sample of children with hemiplegia to study the rate, type and persistence of psychological problems. Most of the rest of this chapter is based on findings of the LHR study, supplemented by clinical experience from our Brain and Behaviour Clinic in the Children's Department of the Maudsley Hospital, London, for the psychological complications of hemiplegia.

In the LHR study, children with hemiplegia were ascertained from multiple sources including hospital and community paediatricians, orthopaedic surgeons, neurosurgeons, hospital and community physiotherapists, special schools and voluntary organisations. A total of 461 individuals under the age of 17 years were recruited from the Greater London area in the UK and all were assessed using parent and teacher questionnaires. Subsequently, 149 of these individuals, all aged between 6 and 10 years, were individually assessed from neurological, psychological and psychiatric perspectives. Judging from demographic, medical, cognitive and behavioural variables, the characteristics of the sample as a whole closely resembled those of previous epidemiological samples of children with hemiplegia (Goodman and Yude 1996). Standardised behavioural screening questionnaires had been completed by the parents and teachers of 428 children who were aged between 2½ and 16 at the time of assessment. The proportion of children scoring above the 'caseness' cut-off on these questionnaires was used to estimate the proportion with psychiatric disorder. Across the entire age band, the proportion with psychiatric disorders was 54% as judged from parental reports and 42% as judged by the reports of teachers or other preschool professionals; there were no consistent age trends, with rates of disorder being high throughout the preschool period, middle childhood years and teenage years (Goodman and Graham 1996). A questionnaire follow up, carried out an average of 4 years later, found that around 70% of children thought to have psychiatric disorders initially were still scoring within the disorder range at follow up (Goodman 1998).

Although the questionnaire findings from the LHR study suggest a high rate of psychiatric disorder throughout childhood, questionnaires are best seen as 'quick-and-dirty' assessment tools whose findings need to be confirmed by detailed individual assessments. When such assessments were carried out on 6 to 10 year olds from the LHR sample, 61% were judged to have at least one diagnosable psychiatric disorder (Goodman and Graham 1996). Common types of disorders included anxiety or depressive disorders in 25% of children; conduct disorders, characterised by disruptive and irritable behaviour, in 24% of children; severe hyperactivity and inattention in 10% of children; and autistic disorders in 3% of children. Some children had more than one type of disorder, with hyperactivity and conduct disorders often occurring together. The common and rare types of disorders are described in more detail in the subsequent sections. Although the LHR study did not involve a control group of children without any physical disability, the overall rate of psychiatric disorder in children with hemiplegia was probably at least three times higher than in children without a physical disability; hyperactivity and autistic disorders were particularly overrepresented.

Fears and worries

Many children with hemiplegia meet the diagnostic criteria for at least one anxiety disorder, with the commonest disorders being specific phobias, separation anxiety and generalised anxiety. While many ordinary children are scared of particular things or situations, specific phobias go beyond this in that the fear results in marked and frequent distress or avoidance, leading to significant curtailment of the child's ordinary life. Some of the specific phobias are exaggerations of common fears, for example, of dogs, heights, injections, lifts, aeroplanes, clowns. In other cases, the phobic stimulus is more unusual, e.g. fluffy things, the sound of coughing, or the smell of oranges. These may not seem very significant but imagine how restricted your life would be if you could never visit friends or relatives without checking that they did not have a fluffy carpet, they did not have a cough, or that there were no oranges around. If you were too embarrassed to ask and put up with the ridicule that would result, you might choose hardly ever to go out. Even staying at home might become very stressful as other family members asserted their right to eat oranges, wear fluffy pullovers, or cough.

Children with hemiplegia, like most children, are particularly attached to one person or to a few key people, looking to these attachment figures for security and turning to them when distressed. Obviously parents are particularly likely to be attachment figures. Although it is normal for children to worry to some degree about being separated from their attachment figures, this can sometimes be so pronounced and impairing that it warrants a diagnosis of separation anxiety disorder. Affected children may insist on sticking close to their parents at all times, following them around from room to room, and resenting being shut outside the toilet door. These children may find it hard to tolerate leaving their parents behind to go to school, getting into a blind panic if their parents are even a few minutes late picking them up after school. It may be impossible for them to go on school outings, to go to Cubs or Brownies, or to go to other children's parties. The intense separation anxiety of some children with hemiplegia is a major problem for them, causing them distress and restricting their lives. In addition, it can be a major burden for the key attachment figure, commonly the mother, who can come to feel like a prisoner who is under constant surveillance.

Generalised anxiety disorder involves substantial distress or social disability occasioned by frequent worries on many topics. These worries can interfere with sleep and concentration and can be associated with prominent physical symptoms such as stomach pains or headaches.

Misery

Many children with hemiplegia feel miserable at times, which is understandable given the difficulties they have to surmount: their physical disability, any associated learning difficulties or teasing and so on. In some cases this misery amounts to a depressive disorder in which markedly and persistently low mood is accompanied by disrupted sleep and appetite, loss of interest and energy, feelings of worthlessness and hopelessness, and suicidal thoughts or behaviours.

Difficult behaviour

The diagnostic terms 'oppositional-defiant disorder' and 'conduct disorder' cover three main types of difficult behaviour: defiant and negativistic behaviour; aggressive behaviour;

and antisocial behaviour such as stealing, robbing or fire-setting. Children with hemiplegia do commonly show markedly defiant and negativistic behaviour, often beginning with severe and frequent temper tantrums at an early age, and continuing with marked irritability throughout childhood accompanied by a great reluctance to do as they are told. On some occasions, these traits can lead to marked aggression, for example, hitting people and throwing things in the course of a temper outburst. This sort of aggression is not the sort of deliberate aggression shown by bullies; it is sometimes described as irritable aggression as opposed to instrumental aggression. In ordinary child mental health clinics, professionals are used to seeing irritability and defiance going along with antisocial behaviour. Fortunately, this is rarely the case in children with hemiplegia, who are very unlikely to enter upon the 'delinquent way of life'. The irritability and oppositionality of so many children with hemiplegia is, perhaps, akin to the way we are all more liable to be short-tempered and uncooperative when deprived of sleep or sickening for something.

Inattention and overactivity

Many children with hemiplegia have their lives, and particularly their education, curtailed by a mixture of fidgetiness, restlessness, poor concentration and easy distractibility. Typically, they will only spend a few minutes on any one task before breaking off to do something else. Even when they are doing something, this is often accompanied by a lot of wriggling, fidgeting, standing up and sitting down. They typically have difficulty staying seated for an entire meal, and often wander off on outings. True hyperactivity and inattention is evident to both parents and teachers. Three diagnostic pitfalls need to be avoided. First, hyperactive children are sometimes surprisingly able to stay still and concentrate for the duration of a brief clinic visit, perhaps because it is interesting and novel, or perhaps because they are overawed by the clinician. Consequently, it is important not to rule out hyperactivity on the basis of what might be a very atypical sample of behaviour in the clinic. A second pitfall is that children often concentrate poorly on things that they do not enjoy or cannot understand. Consequently, a child with dyslexic problems may well seem very restless and inattentive in the classroom because learning is such a trial. The parents may also complain that the child is restless and inattentive when homework has to be done. The clue that this is not true hyperactivity is that the child concentrates well for long periods when doing the sorts of things that he or she is good at, such as building models or drawing. A third and related pitfall is that children with autistic features are often described as hyperactive but this is generally because they are not willing to concentrate for long on activities chosen for them by other people. Once again, the key question is whether they are able to concentrate well when doing something that they have chosen for themselves. Persistence with computer games is not necessarily a good indication of attentional skills since fast-changing games can often keep the attention of children who are otherwise very distractible and impersistent.

Autism and autistic features

Autistic disorders such as infantile autism and Asperger syndrome only affect around 3% of children with hemiplegia, though this is some 10 times higher than the rate of similar disorders in the non-disabled population. By comparison with the relative rarity of full-blown autism, a considerably larger number of children with hemiplegia have some autistic features. Of the children referred to our Brain and Behaviour Clinic for the psychological complications of hemiplegia, roughly a fifth have prominent autistic features. These commonly involve intense preoccupations, some of which are an exaggeration of ordinary childhood interests, for example, a focus on specific cartoon characters to the exclusion of everything else. In other cases, the preoccupation is with an unusual topic such as washing machines, lawn mowers or yogurt pots. These preoccupations are often associated with impoverished pretend play. Some of these children do not engage in any pretend play at all, but the majority do sometimes play out the same simple scenarios over and over again with little variation. Difficulties in social understanding are often shown by a lack of interest in other children or by clumsy attempts to join in with other children, frequently involving telling the other children what to do and not being willing to follow their lead. Delay and deviance in language development is a characteristic part of full-blown autistic syndromes but it is relatively uncommon in children with hemiplegia.

Other psychiatric disorders

A few children with hemiplegia develop obsessions and compulsions, often involving checking things such as electric switches or doing things to avoid contamination, such as repeated hand washing. These obsessions and compulsions are often part of broader anxiety or depressive disorder.

Anorexia nervosa does affect a small number of individuals with hemiplegia, mostly teenage girls. The rate is sufficiently low that it may simply be a coincidence that the same individual has both hemiplegia and an eating disorder. Anecdotally, though, it is possible that the disturbance in body image is partly related to the visuospatial problems that are so common in hemiplegia. Anorexic individuals typically see themselves as fat even when other people think they are far too thin. Perhaps this is more likely to happen to individuals whose visuospatial problems make it very hard to judge the volume of anything, whether it is glass or a box or their own body.

Psychotic illnesses, involving hallucinations or delusions, seem extremely rare. This is both fortunate and theoretically interesting, given that some other childhood neurological disorders are associated with an increased risk of psychotic problems (Ounsted et al. 1987).

Mind-reading skills

Over recent years, developmental psychologists have become increasingly interested in the way children acquire the ability to understand another person's point of view and predict what another person will be feeling or thinking. This is sometimes described in terms of the child developing a 'theory of mind', but it is important to realise that this is primarily a question of being 'on the same wavelength' as other people, which is more an intuitive knack than an intellectual theory. There is increasingly good evidence that children with autism have particular difficulties with mind-reading skills (Happé 1994). Consequently, we predicted that children with hemiplegia and autistic features would have particular problems with mind-reading skills. In fact children with hemiplegia commonly had subtle difficulties with mind-reading skills and many of these children did not seem remotely autistic though they were characterised as emotionally and socially immature by their families and others (Balleny 1996). Typically, these immature children tended to play with younger children or seek out the company of adults, finding it far harder to relate to children of their own age. Their parents often described them as naive in interpersonal relationships and unable to 'read between the lines' in stories and television dramas; they were be able to follow the outline of the plot but found it harder than younger siblings to make sense of irony, deceit or other situations where people meant something rather different from what they said or did. It is not difficult to imagine that difficulty deciphering these sorts of situations will make it much harder for children to participate on equal terms in the fast-moving social world of the playground.

Teasing, bullying, friendship and popularity

The LHR study looked in detail at the peer relationships of a representative sample of 9 to 10 year olds with hemiplegia in mainstream school. By comparison with their classmates, the children with hemiplegia were twice as likely to be rejected, twice as likely to have no friend, and three times as likely to be victimised (Yude et al. 1998). It was very striking that this excess of peer problems occurred in a group whose age and circumstances might have been expected to favour social integration – they were generally in stable peer groups where they had been with the same classmates for 5 years or more. Not all the excess of peer relationship problems could be attributed to learning and behavioural difficulties. The constitutional difficulties in social understanding described in the previous section probably also played a part. Children's prejudices against classmates with disabilities may also be relevant, and in this respect, children with relatively mild physical disabilities may be worse off than children with severe physical disabilities – the latter are more likely to have appropriate allowances made for them, while children with milder disabilities are often unfairly expected to compete on entirely equal terms.

What causes psychiatric problems?

The fact that children with neurological disorders have a higher rate of emotional, behavioural and social difficulties reflects the operation both of organic factors and of psychosocial factors (Goodman 1994). Since the brain is the organ of thought and feeling as well as the organ of movement and perception, it is not surprising that disorders of the brain can directly affect thoughts and feelings as well movements and perceptions. Equally, it is important not to lose sight of how stressful it can be in our society to be physically disabled and experience teasing or school failure due to unrecognised specific learning difficulties. In many cases, organic and psychosocial factors are likely to combine and interact in causing psychiatric problems.

In the LHR study, a higher rate of psychiatric disorder was associated with more severe hemiplegia, some degree of bilateral involvement, the presence of seizures and lower IQ. All of these variables were highly correlated with one another, but in multivariate analyses IQ was the most powerful predictor, with the other variables adding nothing extra once IQ had been allowed for. The most likely explanation for this is that IQ is a particularly sensitive index of the amount of underlying cerebral damage (Goodman and Graham 1996).

The psychiatric problems of children with hemiplegia are associated with a higher rate of parental anxiety and depression and with more parental criticism of the child (Goodman and Graham 1996). Longitudinal studies suggest that this association primarily occurs because the child's problems impose a stress on parents rather than because family stresses cause the child's problems (Goodman 1998). This is not to argue that the child's environment is unimportant, but it is our clinical experience that children's emotional or behavioural difficulties are more likely to arise from stresses in the classroom or playground than from stresses in the home. Indeed, it is commonly the case that children with hemiplegia find the academic and social environment at school very stressful but remain well behaved at school, letting out their frustration and distress on family members once they return home. This can easily mislead the unwary into attributing the child's problems to family stresses. One clue that outbursts at home are fuelled by school stresses is that the child is much better during the school holidays – whereas more contact with the family might be expected to make children's problems worse if the stress originated from home.

One of the potential interests in studying children with hemiplegia is the possibility of comparing children with left- and right-sided hemiplegias, thereby providing a window on the differential specialisation of the two hemispheres. Although various studies of small and unrepresentative groups of children with hemiplegia have claimed side-specific differences in the rate or type of psychiatric problems, this has not been confirmed by studies of large and representative samples (Goodman and Yude 1997). For clinicians and parents, the main implication is that the side of hemiplegia is irrelevant as far as psychological complications are concerned. For the theoretician, the main implication is that the neuroplasticity unleashed by early brain lesions is sufficiently powerful to override any preexisting difference between the two hemispheres. Indeed, it is possible that some of the adverse psychological consequences of early brain damage stem from neuroplasticity, reflecting the adverse effects of new but maladaptive neuronal connections formed in response to the early injury (Goodman 1989).

Treatment

This section is based primarily on our experience treating around 150 children with the psychological complications of hemiplegia. Since the LHR study was an epidemiological rather than an intervention study, it did not provide much information about treatment other than that the great majority of children with hemiplegia and associated psychiatric disorders get no treatment at all. In part, this may simply mirror the fact that most children with psychiatric problems get no help, whether or not they have hemiplegia. In addition, both paediatricians and child psychiatrists sometimes feel out of their depth dealing with problems that cross the brain–behaviour divide. Fortunately, child mental health professionals can be reassured that treating the psychological complications of hemiplegia is mostly similar to their normal work with other children. One difference is that the families of children with hemiplegia are often easier to engage and help than the average family referred to child mental health services. Hemiplegia affects a random cross-section of families (see Introduction) and is not particularly associated with the sorts of family disruption and social disadvantage that are so familiar to child mental health professionals. In addition, the families of children with hemiplegia have long been in contact with paediatric services and are generally willing to accept the advice of well-informed professionals.

When planning psychological treatment, the fact that the child also has hemiplegia does make some difference in four main respects. First, in a society where parents are generally held to be responsible for their children's behaviour problems, it is not surprising that the parents of children with hemiplegia generally feel they must be to blame if their child also develops emotional or behavioural problems. Friends, relatives and even professionals sometimes reinforce this. It is often a great relief to parents to learn that the main cause of their child's behavioural problems is the hemiplegia itself (or rather the same underlying brain disorder that has caused the hemiplegia). Working with many children with hemiplegia, we find it uncanny how often we hear almost identical accounts of behavioural difficulties occurring in very different families. The families themselves are often fascinated and relieved to hear this. Further relief comes from sharing experiences directly with other families through newsletters and meetings (see chapter 14). Knowing that emotional and behavioural difficulties have biological origins is obviously not an excuse for doing nothing about them. Parents and professionals sometimes fall into the trap of assuming that because the underlying brain disorder is irreversible, nothing can be done about the psychological consequences. Yet just as physiotherapy or antiepileptic medication can reduce or eliminate some of the physical consequences of the brain disorder, so appropriate treatment can reduce or eliminate the psychological complications. Reducing unnecessary guilt by emphasising the role of brain–behaviour links need not be at the cost of abandoning other forms of treatment.

A second respect in which the presence of hemiplegia may influence the treatment of psychological complications is that it is sometimes essential to focus not on the behaviour but on the child's epilepsy. When the child has behavioural problems and poorly controlled epilepsy, improving seizure control through changes in medication or surgery (see chapters 10 and 11) is often accompanied by a dramatic improvement in behaviour. On occasions, the child's behaviour is also worsened by a particular antiepileptic medication, with parents usually having noticed that the behavioural difficulties have waxed and waned as the dose of a particular antiepileptic medication has altered. Barbiturates used to be common culprits, but nowadays it is more common to see behavioural worsening associated with benzodiazepines, sodium valproate or vigabatrin, though any antiepileptic medication can be responsible at times. On occasions, frequent ultra-brief epileptic discharges (transient cognitive impairments) can mimic the attention difficulties seen in hyperactivity. EEGs are not normally needed when assessing the psychological complications of hemiplegia, but they are sometimes indicated if the history or direct observation suggests the child's attention is often interrupted by what could be frequent brief seizures.

Hemiplegia can also be relevant to the treatment of psychological complications in a third way if the affected individual, commonly in the teenage years, is tacitly or explicitly denying the physical disability. Particularly if the hemiplegia is mild, the teenager may refuse to acknowledge it or accept the sort of help needed to circumvent it. For example, hemiplegia plus some degree of involvement of the 'good' side can make writing extremely difficult, in which case regular access to a laptop computer in school can make an enormous difference

– but some teenagers refuse to accept this because it would make them look different from their classmates and they prefer to be 'ordinary failures' who write a few illegible lines with difficulty rather than being successes who openly acknowledge a potential disability and then circumvent it. It is not easy to get round teenagers' understandable desire to 'be one of the crowd', but their failure to acknowledge their disability often buys temporary relief at the cost of greater long-term stress.

The fourth point is the inverse of the previous point. If failure to accept appropriate help for circumventing hemiplegia can sometimes lead to worsened stress and adverse psychological consequences, so too can the imposition of inappropriate help for hemiplegia. For example, inappropriately intense physiotherapy programmes may consume much of the child's time without corresponding benefit (see chapter 6). Apart from wasting time the child could otherwise be spending with friends or getting on with age-appropriate activities, this also builds up resentment towards parents and professionals.

After allowing for these factors that are relatively specific to hemiplegia or related conditions, the treatment for emotional, attention or behavioural difficulties makes use of the same specific techniques that are employed in child mental health practice in general (Goodman and Scott 1997). The main features of these approaches are summarised in the following sections.

Treatment of attention deficit and hyperactivity
Severe and pervasive attention deficit with hyperactivity often responds well to stimulant medication. Methylphenidate is usually the treatment of choice, but some clinicians prefer to use dexamphetamine in children who also have seizures. Treatment with stimulant medication is unlikely to be helpful for the child whose inattention is due to frequent unrecognised seizures, or for the child who concentrates well on favourite activities. When children do have attentional difficulties, it is vital that their teaching takes this into account, with new concepts being broken down into subcomponents that can be mastered within the child's attention span, and with frequent repetition subsequently to consolidate the learning. If parents and teachers can recognise the child's distractible and restless behaviour as something that is largely beyond the child's control, and not a sign of laziness or badness, it is easier to avoid the constant criticism and character assassination that can fuel resentment and associated behavioural problems.

Treating oppositional and defiant problems
Children who are constitutionally particularly hard to manage need 'superparents' and 'superteachers' to control and contain them. Providing additional parent training or classroom management training can be helpful even though these parents and teachers have often been extremely good at bringing up and teaching less challenging children. Successful behavioural approaches generally involve consistency, praise and other rewards for desirable behaviours, and immediate but brief sanctions for negative behaviours (for example, 2 minutes of 'time-out' for non-compliance with a previous request). While all children need to learn to cope with some frustrations and comply with adult requests, it is often helpful where possible to avoid unnecessary stresses and frictions. Expecting the child to be perfectly behaved on all

occasions is a recipe for failure, nagging and stress for all concerned, whereas concentrating rewards and sanctions on a few key behaviours can be far more successful. Both at home and at school, it can be helpful to provide an 'asylum' for children to retreat to when they know they are losing control. This may be the child's bedroom at home, or an office or sick room at school. If the child can be helped to recognise when they are becoming overwrought, so that they can go off and calm down for a few minutes, this can avert an explosion (and the ensuing row) that would otherwise have overshadowed the whole day. In our experience, children do not usually abuse their right to seek asylum. Finally, it is important to remember that the constitutional irritability of many children with hemiplegia is often considerably worsened by environmental stresses. These stresses typically originate in school, often as a result of unrecognised learning difficulties, inadequate help with these difficulties, victimisation by classmates, or lack of friends. If these stresses can be reduced, the child often becomes more compliant and less prone to temper outbursts.

Treating emotional problems

The appropriate treatment for phobias is nearly always desensitization. With explanation and encouragement, children will usually agree to being exposed, not to the thing they fear most, but to a related stimulus that they fear only slightly. For example, someone who fears touching fluffy things might agree to begin touching a smooth fabric and gradually work up towards velvet. They may then be willing to touch increasingly fluffy materials until finally, perhaps after many graded sessions, they are willing to touch the sorts of fluffy jumpers, carpets or toys that they previously avoided. Much of the exposure is done as 'homework', often with the help of trusted family members, rather than in sessions with the therapist. Much of the skill of therapy lies in finding a sufficient number of intermediate stages so that children never have to tackle anything that they find more than very mildly anxiety provoking. Separation anxiety is treated in a rather similar way, gradually training the child to cope with progressively longer separations from key attachment figures. For example, the mother may help a child play round at a friend's home by staying there throughout on the first occasion. On the subsequent occasion, when the child is well settled, he or she may agree to the mother going away for 5 minutes, perhaps to get something for the child from the shops. (If the child has little sense of time, it can be reassuring to set a kitchen timer to 5 minutes so that the child can easily see how much time is left.) On further occasions, the length of time the mother is away can gradually be extended. As with all other desensitisation techniques, the child's tolerance of previously feared situations is gradually increased without pushing so hard that the child becomes overwhelmed. Generalised anxiety can be tackled using relaxation techniques or by teaching children 'self talk' so that they can reassure themselves and generate the strategies they need for combating stress. When children are depressed, the most successful strategy is often to tackle the contributory stresses, mostly in the school situation. In some severely depressed teenagers, treatment with selective serotonin reuptake inhibitors (SSRIs) can be helpful. SSRIs can also be useful, along with behavioural therapy, for obsessions and compulsions. Medication is generally not indicated for anxiety disorders, with the possible exception of panic attacks.

Autistic problems

Autistic disorders and lesser autistic features are relatively enduring, so it is important not to aim for unrealistic goals. Since the child is unlikely to change dramatically or rapidly, it is all the more important to alter both the child's environment and the expectations of family and teachers. Behavioural approaches that are designed to reduce unwanted behaviours or encourage desired behaviours can be useful provided they are not over ambitious. One of the difficulties in designing such programmes is finding suitable rewards. Children with autistic features are less concerned about what other people think and feel and, therefore, are far less amenable to social pressures and rewards. Eliminating unusual interests such as fiddling with bits of string, may be unrealistic; restricting these activities to certain times of day may be more workable. Indeed, it may be possible to use permission to engage briefly in these activities as a reward for doing ordinary household or classroom activities. It is sometimes possible to harness a tendency to ritualise activities to beneficial ends for example, establishing a 'getting-ready-for-school' or a 'getting-ready-for-bed' ritual. Patience is vital, as is consistency over time, and consistency between home and school. Indeed, residential schooling is sometimes particularly valuable for these children because a well-resourced and skilled school can sometimes provide dispassionate 24-hour consistency that cannot be expected of any family.

Adult outcome

The LHR has followed up children and teenagers with hemiplegia into early adult life. The preliminary results are guardedly encouraging (Goodman et al. 1998). Although children with hemiplegia have a high rate of psychiatric disorder, their rate of psychiatric illness in adulthood does not seem to be particularly raised (though severe autistic disorders do generally persist). While it is encouraging that young adults with life-long hemiplegia do not seem to be at particularly high risk of anxiety disorders, depression or schizophrenia, this is only part of the story. In some instances, childhood difficulties with emotional and behavioural problems persist as maladaptive and restricting personality traits that interfere with the quality of the individual's life in adulthood, even if these traits are not classified as a psychiatric illness. While many young adults with hemiplegia lead full and fulfilling lives, others lead unnecessarily restricted lives. Sometimes, this is due to the individual's tendency to withdraw from social situations, perhaps in continuity with earlier separation anxiety. In other instances, earlier irritability and negativism lead on to an abrasive personality style that makes it hard to form and keep friendships. Far too many individuals leave school to live out a very constrained life in the family home, with few opportunities for fulfillment through work, friendships or leisure activities. This is not a necessary consequence of hemiplegia, even when the hemiplegia is associated with additional problems such as epilepsy or learning difficulties. With appropriate help, some individuals with severe hemiplegia and several associated problems are living fulfilling adult lives. Nevertheless, the fact that this is not universal emphasises the need for early help when it is called for, and for an education that progressively builds up social and self-help skills in order to prepare each individual for an adult life that is as independent and fulfilling as possible.

REFERENCES

Balleny, H. (1996) *Are the Concepts of 'Theory of Mind' and 'Executive Function' Useful in Understanding Social Impairment in Children with Hemiplegic CP?* Clin Psy D thesis. University of East Anglia, Norwich.

Breslau, N. (1985) Psychiatric disorder in children with physical disabilities. *Journal of the American Academy of Child Psychiatry*, **24**, 87–94.

Goodman, R. (1989) Neuronal misconnections and psychiatric disorder: Is there a link? *British Journal of Psychiatry*, **154**, 292–299.

— (1994) Brain Disorders. *In:* Rutter, M., Taylor, E., Hersov, L. (Eds.) *Child and Adolescent Psychiatry, 3rd Edn.* Oxford: Blackwell Scientific Publications, p. 172–190.

— (1998) The longitudinal stability of psychiatric problems in children with hemiplegia. *Journal of Child Psychology and Psychiatry*, **39**, 347–54.

— Graham, P. (1996) Psychiatric problems in children with hemiplegia: cross sectional epidemiological survey. *British Medical Journal*, **312**, 1065–1069.

— Yude, C. (1996) Do incomplete ascertainment and recruitment matter? *Developmental Medicine and Child Neurology*, **38**, 156–165.

— Scott, S. (1997) *Child Psychiatry*. Oxford: Blackwell Science.

— Yude, C. (1997) Do unilateral lesions of the developing brain have side-specific psychiatric consequences in childhood? *Laterality*, **2**, 103–115.

— O'Neill, T., Beecham, J. (1998) *Provision for individuals with hemiplegic cerebral palsy: What happens when they outgrow children's services. A final report for the NHS Executive.* Available from the NHS or the authors of this chapter.

Happé, F.G.E. (1994) Current psychological theories of autism: the 'Theory of Mind' account and rival theories. *Journal of Child Psychology and Psychiatry*, **35**, 215–229.

Ingram, T.T.S. (1955) A study of cerebral palsy in the childhood population of Edinburgh. *Archives of Disease in Childhood*, **30**, 8598.

— (1956) A characteristic form of overactive behaviour in brain damaged children. *Journal of Mental Science*, **102**, 550–558.

Krynauw, R.A. (1950) Infantile hemiplegia treated by removing one cerebral hemisphere. *Journal of Neurology, Neurosurgery and Psychiatry*, **13**, 243–267.

Ounsted, C. (1955) The hyperkinetic syndrome in epileptic children. *Lancet*, **ii**, 303–311.

— Lindsay, J., Richards, P. (1987) *Temporal Lobe Epilepsy 1948–1986: A Biographical Study. Clinics in Developmental Medicine No. 103.* London: Mac Keith Press.

Rutter, M., Graham, P., Yule, W. (1970) *A Neuropsychiatric Study in Childhood. Clinics in Developmental Medicine Nos. 35/36.* London: Spastics International Medical Publications.

Seidel, U.P., Chadwick, O.F.D., Rutter, M. (1975) Psychological disorders in crippled children. A comparative study of children with and without brain damage. *Developmental Medicine and Child Neurology*, **17**, 563–573.

Uvebrant, P. (1988) Hemiplegic cerebral palsy aetiology and outcome. *Acta Paediatrica Scandinavica*, **Suppl. 345**, 1–100.

Yude, C., Goodman R., McConachie, H. (1998) Peer problems of children with hemiplegia in mainstream primary schools. *Journal of Child Psychology and Psychiatry*, **39**, 533–41.

13
NEUROPSYCHOLOGY AND EDUCATIONAL MANAGEMENT

Valerie Muter and Faraneh Vargha-Khadem

When lateralised brain injury occurs in adults, there is selective loss of previously intact cognitive functions resulting in clinical conditions such as aphasia, amnesia, alexia and so on (Shallice 1988, McCarthy and Warrington 1990). Such syndromes have highlighted the modular nature of adult cognitive functioning. There is, however, clear recognition that the cognitive sequelae of injuries sustained in infancy or early childhood are very different from those acquired in adulthood or even later childhood. The aim of this chapter is, first, to consider briefly theoretical frameworks in cognitive neuropsychology which attempt to explain issues relevant to the impact of pre- and perinatal injury. Second, we aim to review evidence from neuropsychological studies of childhood hemiplegia, with particular emphasis on the language and educational consequences of lateralised damage and finally, to examine the implications for assessment and teaching of children with hemiplegia.

Some cognitive neuropsychologists have argued that, in contrast to the findings in adults, the evidence in children points to specific cognitive modules becoming gradually established over time, with aspects of learning required for their delineation. Karmiloff-Smith (1992) proposes that "..nature specifies initial biases or predispositions that channel attention to relevant environmental inputs, which in turn affect subsequent brain development ... development involves a process of gradual modularisation" (p. 5). Thus, a major issue in cognitive neuropsychology concerns the ways in which disordered development impinges upon the process of gradual modularisation (Temple 1997).

A rather different perspective draws on neural network and connectionist models (see Plunkett et al. 1997, for a review). Specifically, in relation to language development, Bates (1992) has proposed that "there is enormous plasticity in the brain regions that can support language ... and the areas responsible for language learning are not necessarily the same regions that mediate use and maintenance of language in adults" (p. 182). She goes on to conclude that language learning is not highly 'domain specific' but is instead based on a relatively plastic mix of neural systems that also serve other functions. Plasticity, a central concept of developmental neuropsychology, may be explained in neural network terms as follows: regions with particular computational resources i.e. those with the necessary architectural bias for language are recruited for language tasks. If these units are not available due to a focal lesion, then other regions of the neural network with access to relevant inputs are recruited instead. Although these units may not be as architecturally refined for language function as the original damaged regions, they nonetheless are usually able to take over the task, often performing at or only slightly below normal levels, depending on the particular language skill. Vargha-Khadem (1993) goes on to discuss the mechanisms of plasticity and progressive lateralisation as working in opposition to each other during childhood. When a lateralised lesion is incurred early, then it is lateralisation of function that is sacrificed to reorganisation processes made possible by the plasticity of the young brain. For lesions sustained later in life, lateralisation becomes progressively more prominent and plasticity is reduced, with the result that increasingly specific cognitive deficits arise from a localised cerebral insult. Additionally, the loss of a degree of overall intellectual 'power' following early focal injury is thought to be a cost of the successful reorganisation of language function (Hebb 1942); in effect, greater neuronal 'power' is needed to initiate and develop a cognitive function than is needed to maintain it once it is established. Hence, there is a general lowering of overall cognitive ability following early injury which is not evident in adult-sustained injuries.

Equipotentiality, functional reorganisation and cognitive crowding
A major concept in developmental cognitive neuropsychology that has particular implications for children with congenital hemiplegia is that of equipotentiality. Lenneberg (1967) suggested that at birth the two cerebral hemispheres are equipotential for language function. The hemispheres become progressively specialised during the course of childhood until about the age of 12 years after which their functions become crystallised, closely resembling the adult form of hemispheric specialisation.

The research literature has produced conflicting results in respect of the equipotentiality hypothesis which has had an interesting history (for a more comprehensive appraisal of the literature, see Vargha-Khadem et al. 1994). In the 1970s and 1980s, evidence accumulated that anatomic, electrophysiological and functional asymmetries typical of adults could also be demonstrated in young children (supporting the 'antiequipotentiality' stance). However, there has been in the late 1980s and early 1990s a renewal of interest in a modified form of the equipotentiality hypothesis. This has been prompted by the increased availability of fine-grained data from large-scale studies, and by the greater awareness of (often previously uncontrolled) factors that can significantly affect cognitive outcome: these include unsuspected bilateral pathology, presence of seizures and use of anticonvulsant medication, stage of development of the cognitive function under study, age at onset of lesion, time elapsed since onset of lesion, and age at testing (for a fuller discussion of these variables see Vargha-Khadem et al. 1994). Recognising that neither early specialisation nor equipotentiality could serve as useful constructs if they were regarded as absolutes, Satz and colleagues (1990) have argued for a continuum, with equipotentiality and early specialisation occupying the two extremes. More recent research has tended to favour the equipotentiality end of the continuum.

Vargha-Khadem and coworkers (1992) studied IQ and memory function in a series of 82 hemiplegic children with congenital damage, and found no evidence to support the early specialisation position. The group without seizures was impaired relative to normal control subjects on Performance IQ scores only, and not on any aspect of verbal or memory function. However, when the patients with seizures were compared to the non-seizure patients and the control group, the former were impaired on all measures of IQ and almost all measures of verbal and non-verbal memory. Thus, a decrement in the level of general cognitive skill would appear to be a consequence of interference caused by seizures and/or medication. Similar results were obtained in studies by Carlsson et al. (1994), Goodman and Yude (1996) and Muter et al. (1997). However, Goodman and Yude (1996) have suggested that there are other neurological factors, in addition to seizures, which may influence degree of cognitive impairment. In their sample of 149 children with hemiplegia assessed neurologically and psychometrically, 53% of the variance in the scores of the Weschler Intelligence Scale for Children-Revised (WISC-R, Weschler 1976) was accounted for by five neurological variables which together formed an 'N score' i.e. age at onset, severity, bilateral involvement, seizure history and head circumference. The authors suggest that a neurological index such as this might function as a useful alternative or adjunct to developmental tests when predicting eventual IQ in very young children with hemiplegia (particularly those under the age of 3 years).

Recent findings support the view that either hemisphere has the ability to subserve verbal functions in the face of early unilateral damage. The observation of a lowered performance IQ irrespective of side of injury is in accord with the notion of cognitive crowding proposed by Teuber (1975). Language skills are preserved in the early injured brain, irrespective of side of injury, through a process of reorganisation within the remaining intact regions. However, this preservation may be achieved at the expense of other aspects of cognitive functioning, in particular visuospatial skills. In the case of a left-hemisphere injury, language skills are prioritised in the competition for neural space, and so are effectively spared, at least at a gross level. However, to accommodate this reorganisation, other skills are assigned a lower order of priority, and their development is rendered deficient. In the case of a right-hemisphere injury, the selective lowering of the performance IQ is a direct consequence of damage to those regions specialised for visuospatial processing. Carlsson and coworkers (1994) have suggested that there is a difference between the sexes in the ability to reorganise language functions following early focal injury. They found that the verbal functioning of girls in their group with an injured left hemisphere was significantly more impaired than that of the boys; they propose that boys reorganise verbal skills more completely to the right hemisphere, thus implying a larger 'crowding' effect on non-verbal function. However, the studies by Goodman and Yude (1996) and Muter and colleagues (1997) failed to confirm this effect of sex.

Cognitive skills and their stability in congenital hemiplegia

In general, most studies of children with focal brain injury report lower Full-Scale IQ scores when compared to control subjects (see Bates et al. 1999, and Vargha-Khadem et al. 1994, for reviews); the group difference between brain-injured and normal control subjects is relatively small, although the range of IQs within the population with focal lesions is very large, ranging from those with learning disabilities through to those who perform well above average.

Banich and colleagues (1990) found in a cross-sectional study of children with congenital hemiplegia that the longer the time elapsed since lesion onset, the lower the level of intellectual functioning. This suggests that children with hemiplegia may show a slowing down in their rate of cognitive growth as they get older. However, this study might be criticised, first, for its inclusion of children with very low ability whose diverse injuries implicated possibly diffuse damage, and second, the failure to take account of seizure status. A longitudinal study of cognitive function in children with hemiplegia which employed standardised IQ tests is that reported by Aram and Eisele (1994). They obtained Wechsler IQ scores from 26 patients with unilateral lesions at two points in time. Their results revealed normal levels of intellectual performance with relatively minor decrements in IQ over time, and then associated only with right-hemisphere injury.

The findings from our own longitudinal study of 38 children tested on the Wechsler Intelligence Scales (Wechsler 1963, 1976) between the ages of 4 and 6 years (Muter et al. 1997) are in agreement with the findings of Aram and Eisele. The children with hemiplegia in our study all showed stability of their IQ scores over the study period. However, one caution should be borne in mind; the children participating in our research were comparatively young and were followed up for only 2 years in all. The selection of a young sample of subjects necessarily restricts the range and complexity of skills that may be studied. In these subjects, gross verbal and non-verbal abilities appeared to be well established, but some of the more subtle and complex aspects of language function thought to develop at a later age could not be evaluated. Banich and colleagues (1990) and Goldman (1974) have suggested that the reorganisational capacity of the young damaged brain is adequate to support early developing functions but not more complex functions (for instance, metacognitive and educational skills) that would be expected to develop later as the brain matures. In the following sections, we will review studies that have highlighted selective deficits in language and educational skills after unilateral damage. It may be the case that unilaterally brain-damaged children need to be evaluated over a longer period of time and well into later childhood in order to observe the decline in cognitive function which Banich and colleagues (1990) and Goldman (1974) have proposed.

Language skills in children with hemiplegia
The evidence reviewed thus far points to gross language skills being remarkably well preserved in children with hemiplegia whose injury has been sustained pre- or perinatally. However, it appears that, not only do visuospatial skills become deficient as a result of functional reorganisation, but the development of specific language abilities may also be impaired. A number of studies investigating selective language deficits in children with congenital hemiplegia support this view.

Studies conducted by Aram and her colleagues in the 1980s and early 1990s have reported that children with early left-sided lateralised injury perform below the levels of matched control subjects on a wide range of specific language tests. In contrast, the language skills of children with early right-sided injury are not markedly different from those of control individuals. Patients with left-sided injury have been found to be specifically impaired in respect of: syntax, vocabulary, naming fluency and phoneme discrimination (Rankin et al. 1981), simple and complex sentence structure (Aram et al. 1986), lexical retrieval (Aram et al. 1987), and comprehension and production of complex grammar (Eisele and Aram 1994).

182

While the evidence pertaining to subtle language deficits in children with left-hemisphere damage appears compelling, methodological considerations demand a more cautious interpretation of these earlier findings (for a critical review, see Bishop 1983, 1988).

Vargha-Khadem and Mishkin (1997) have suggested that, although selective language deficits may be observed in cases of left-hemisphere injury, the level of language skill is nonetheless consistent with overall cognitive ability (which is at least mildly depressed in children with hemiplegia). Consistent with this, Bates and colleagues (1999) have shown that, when IQ is entered as a covariate in analyses of selective language function, many of the reported differences between groups disappear.

More recently, neuropsychological investigations have reported fine-grained studies of language, some within a longitudinal framework. A series of studies of relatively large numbers of children with unilateral lesions has been conducted by Bates and her colleagues (Thal et al. 1997, Reilly et al. 1998, Bates et al. 1999). Thal and coworkers (1997) studied 53 infants and preschool children between the ages of 10 and 44 months. The results from the age range 10 to 17 months suggest that children with right-hemisphere injuries are at greater risk for delays in word comprehension, and in the symbolic and communicative gestures that normally precede and accompany language onset. The authors suggest, that to understand words at this age, children must integrate information from many different sources and modalities; the integrative processes in the right hemisphere may predominate in word comprehension, thus placing children with right-hemisphere injuries at a specific (though apparently temporary) disadvantage.

The capacity of the injured brain to recover function is understandably modified by a range of factors such as age at onset of injury, size and site of the lesion, and the presence of seizures.

Studies of handedness and dichotic listening have thrown light on the relation between size of lesion and reorganisation of language. The intimate relation between hand dominance and the lateralisation of language implies that handedness provides a useful and non-invasive indicator of cerebral lateralisation in clinical populations. If an unusually high incidence of left-handedness is found in children with early left-hemisphere damage, it suggests reorganisation not only of motor but also of language representation. A further behavioural measure of language lateralisation is dichotic listening, which has been used to investigate asymmetry of auditory processing and, by implication, hemispheric functional specialisation (Kimura 1961). In the dichotic listening paradigm, when verbal material is presented to both ears simultaneously, the majority of normal adults and children report more accurately from the right ear, this being indicative of left-hemisphere processing of language (Kimura 1961, Hiscock and Decter 1988). Studies of dichotic listening in patients with unilateral lesions have aimed to investigate the effects of such lesions in altering the normal functional representations of the cerebral hemispheres. Children who have acquired left-hemisphere lesions early in life (at a time when plasticity should permit functional reorganisation) would be expected to show a left-ear advantage if language functions have indeed come to be represented by the right-hemisphere. In support of this, Carlsson and coworkers (1992) found that 78% of their left-hand dominant patients with left-hemisphere injuries (as verified by CT scans) demonstrated a left-ear advantage on a dichotic listening task, in contrast to only 35% of normal left-handers. In a large-scale study of children with hemiplegia, Isaacs and colleagues (1996) showed that the presence of congenital left-hemisphere injury led to an alteration of the normal right-ear advantage. The authors proposed that children showing a marked left-ear advantage were likely to have more extensive left-hemisphere lesions (confirmed by CT scans) that encroached on language-related areas than those in whom the right-ear advantage had been maintained; thus, in the former group there was an enforced transfer of language to the right hemisphere. This finding is compatible with the results of the classic study by Rasmussen and Milner (1977) in which Sodium Amytal investigations of language lateralisation in adults with early left-hemisphere damage were carried out. Injection of the anaesthetic, Sodium Amytal, into one hemisphere of the brain enables the functions of the contralateral hemisphere to be studied separately in the functional absence of the anaesthetised one. They found that right-hemisphere mediation of language was more likely in individuals with larger left-hemisphere lesions involving the perisylvian area.

There is some evidence that size of lesion may have less of an effect on cognitive outcome than presence of seizures. Vargha-Khadem and colleagues (1992) found that the degree of intellectual deficit and verbal memory and learning impairment was highly related to presence of seizure and/or severe EEG abnormality. Unilateral brain damage, even if it was extensive (as verified by CT or MRI scans) resulted in few and only mild deficits, provided the damage was not accompanied by seizure activity or severe EEG abnormality.

There is very little reliable evidence concerning the relation between lesion site and cognitive functioning. Aram and Ekelman (1986) attempted to relate characteristics of the WISC-R profile of their subjects with hemiplegia to the site of lesion. The resultant small groups precluded statistical analysis and only tentative observations were reported. In the study by Levine et al. (1987), no relation was found between lesion site and IQ. Thal and colleagues (1997) investigated the interaction between lesion site and language skill in their sample of infant and preschool children with hemiplegia. These authors have suggested different site-specific effects may be evident at different stages of development, and are dependent on the task in hand. After age 5, these site-specific effects may be difficult to detect indicating that a substantial degree of inter- and/or intrahemispheric reorganisation has taken place.

The specific language skills of our sample studied longitudinally (Muter et al. 1994) were investigated through the administration of a range of standardised and experimental tests that included measures of receptive vocabulary and grammar, word naming, expressive sentence construction and word fluency. IQ was entered as a covariate in all the analyses; this enabled an appraisal of the specific effects of seizures on language performance over and above those explicable in terms of the lower IQ of the seizure groups. In general, the results showed that there were no marked detrimental effects of hemispheric side of injury on language function, other than those that might be accounted for by IQ differences, thus supporting the view that the two hemispheres are equipotential for language processing, at least in the groups without seizures.

However, there was a series of significant results that indicated that one particular group with hemiplegia, namely the left-hemisphere damaged group with seizures had exceptional difficulty in language functioning. This group was impaired relative to both the right-hemisphere group with seizures and the left-hemisphere group without seizures on measures of receptive vocabulary (British Picture Vocabulary Test, Dunn et al. 1982) at age 4 and expressive formulation of sentences (Clinical Evaluation of Language Fundamentals- Revised, CELF-R, Semel et al.1987) at age 5. Children with early hemispheric injury, provided they are seizure free, develop apparently normal language functioning, at least at a gross level. This is true even for children with left-hemisphere insults at least some of whom would be expected to have undergone a substantial degree of language reorganisation. The right hemisphere may, under favourable circumstances, successfully take over language processing, as evidenced by the sparing of function in the seizure-free left-hemisphere group. Although we acknowledge the limitations imposed both by our small sample size and the need for replication within independent studies, we might speculate that seizures interfere with what is usually a successful reorganisation process. An explanation for the foregoing findings draws on dichotic listening data from the left-hemisphere group with seizures. We found that there was a substantially reduced right-ear advantage in the group with left-hemisphere injuries, this being indicative of a tendency towards greater right-hemisphere processing of language. The right-hemisphere shift was especially pronounced in the children with a left-hemisphere insult accompanied by seizures. We suggest that these children must face a double challenge; they need to achieve reorganisation of language function through a shift to right-hemisphere processing and they must cope with the secondary effects of seizure spread and anticonvulsant medication. The children with right-hemisphere damage accompanied by seizures also experience the deleterious consequences of seizures (and medication), but they do not have to undergo the processes of reorganisation and hemispheric shift of language as the left-hemisphere is relatively undamaged.

Educational skills in children with hemiplegia
Few studies have addressed educational and related skills in children with hemiplegia. Clinic-based studies have suggested that children with hemiplegia are at risk for reading and spelling difficulties and also mathematical problems (Dorman 1987 and Haskell 1966, respectively). However, studies such as these are prone to referral bias which may render the sample unrepresentative of the population of children with hemiplegia. An experimental study by Aram and Ekelman (1988) investigated the performance of children with hemiplegia on a standardised educational measure i.e. the Woodcock-Johnson Psychoeducational Battery (1977) which includes literacy and numeracy subtests. The results failed to demonstrate any differences in performance in relation to hemispheric side of injury or any specific patterns of difficulty, although the sample with hemiplegia did score marginally below the matched control individuals on all the subtests.

In contrast, a recent study by Frampton and colleagues (1998) found that, in a representative sample of 59 children with hemiplegia aged between 6 and 10 years, more than one-third qualified as having a specific learning difficulty (in reading, spelling or mathematics), identified on the basis of ability–achievement discrepancies that would put them in the lowest 5% of the population. This prevalence rate for specific learning difficulties is substantially higher than that found in the normal population. The best predictor of the occurrence of a specific learning difficulty was an index of neurological impairment which was generated from age at onset of brain damage, severity of hemiplegia, seizure history, bilateral pathology and reduced head circumference.

In cognitive developmental research conducted over the past 20 years, there has been a very strong emphasis on the causal relation between phonological awareness (the child's sensitivity to speech-sound segments in words) and the facility to learn to read and spell. Phonological skills and their crucial role in launching literacy skills have been extensively studied in normal populations (see Adams 1990, Goswami and Bryant 1990, for reviews), and also in certain clinical populations, notably children suffering from dyslexia. Group and individual case studies have shown that the majority of individuals with dyslexia have poor phonological awareness and consequently find it hard to adopt sequential decoding strategies in reading and spelling (Hulme and Snowling 1992, Rack et al. 1992).

Phonological awareness was investigated longitudinally in the same sample of children with hemiplegia reported earlier by administering tests of rhyming, phoneme blending, phoneme segmentation and phoneme deletion in each of the 3 years of the study (Muter 1994). The presence of a unilateral lesion, irrespective of hemispheric side of lesion or seizure status, had no deleterious effects on phonological awareness, other than those that might be accounted for by IQ. There is, therefore, evidence to suggest that basic phonological skills are preserved in the early injured brain, even when the damage is to the left hemisphere.

The children were also administered tests of reading and spelling at ages 5 and 6 and tests of numeracy at age 6 (Muter et al. 1994). The presence of a unilateral insult, irrespective of the hemispheric side of insult, did not impair literacy or numeracy skills, but in this case only if the injury was not accompanied by seizures. It seems somewhat surprising that the children with hemiplegia did so well in arithmetic, bearing in mind their poor visuospatial skills (see section 'Equipotentiality, functional reorganisation and cognitive crowding'). In fact, the seizure-free group with hemiplegia was making remarkably good educational progress. These findings appear to contradict those of Frampton and coworkers. However, it should be borne in mind that the children in our sample were in general far younger than those in the study by Frampton and colleagues; it may be that children with hemiplegia make a promising beginning in acquiring educational skills, but fail to sustain this rate of progress as they are required to learn more complex academic skills. We also found that the left-hemisphere group with seizures was particularly disadvantaged in reading and arithmetical attainments relative to the left-hemisphere group without seizures (and in arithmetic, relative to the right-hemisphere group with seizures). This was an effect over and above the effects of the lower IQ of the children with seizures. These findings are in accord with those for the language measures and seem to indicate that children with left-hemisphere insult accompanied by seizures are particularly at risk within the hemiplegic population, not only in respect of their spoken language but also their educational development. Frampton and colleagues found a correlation between the likelihood of having a specific learning difficulty and an index of neurological severity in which one of their criteria was the presence of seizures.

Much has been made of the importance of the causal relation between phonology and reading in normally developing children and children with dyslexia. We addressed this question in our groups of seizure-free subjects with hemiplegia through a series of correlational analyses (Muter et al. 1994). We found that the expected correlation between phonology and reading was apparent in the children with right-hemisphere damage, but was much reduced in those with left-hemisphere damage. It is possible that the left hemisphere is uniquely specialised not so much for the development of literacy and phonological skills per se but for subserving their interaction and integration. Thus, the capacity of other regions of the brain, be they inter- or intrahemispheric, to take over these integrative functions, even in the case of early injury, may be somewhat limited.

We also found that the group with left-hemisphere injury showed stronger correlations between letter knowledge and reading and between verbal memory and reading than both the control group and the group with right-hemisphere insult. This suggests that, in the absence of strong phonology–reading connections, children with left-hemisphere damage may be making successful use of alternative skills, specifically letter knowledge and verbal memory, to promote their early reading development. Given the small sample sizes and the relatively large number of statistical analyses conducted, we regard these conclusions as preliminary and speculative. Whether the children with left-hemisphere injury would be able to sustain this good rate of progress, without the support of important phonology–literacy connections, is an issue for further research. In fact, there is evidence that the contribution of phonological processing to reading and spelling may extend beyond the early stages of literacy development to the later stages of learning in primary school (Muter and Snowling 1998). Indeed, the findings from our own study and that of Frampton and coworkers, lead us to suspect that children with hemiplegia may develop more pronounced educational difficulties as they get older. As Reilly and colleagues (1998) have pointed out, in the face of early pathology, recovery should be viewed as a continuing process, with the child having to respond afresh to each new cognitive challenge in ongoing development without the benefit of the substrate that is most usually recruited for that given skill; early focal injury, and the need for ongoing recovery processes exact a lasting price, but the shape of the 'price tag' changes with the stage of development under study and the linguistic challenge at hand.

Conclusions

It is proposed that a unilateral injury, provided that it is incurred early in life and is not accompanied by seizures, produces few detrimental effects on either spoken language or educational skills, at least in the early stages of childhood. Plasticity of the developing brain provides sufficient compensatory mechanisms for effective functional reorganisation within the remaining neural space. This is true even when the injury is in the left hemisphere where damage during adult life results in selective language deficits.

However, our studies have uncovered three limiting factors to successful reorganisation of cognitive function. The influence of such factors results in what Bates and colleagues (1999) refer to as 'constrained plasticity'. Thus, left-hemisphere bias for language involves 'soft' constraints which are both probabilistic in nature – not all-or-none – and are not irreversible and can be overcome. The constraints we identified were, first, the presence of seizures (and possibly other neurological indices) which has a general depressing effect on cognitive function, as measured by IQ tests. Second, left-hemisphere insult accompanied by seizures may result in deficits in receptive and expressive language, and in early reading and numeracy skills, over and above those accounted for by lowered IQ. While this novel finding clearly requires replication, we might speculate that, in the presence of a left-hemisphere injury, seizures appear to disrupt the capacity of the right hemisphere to successfully subserve language processing. Third, a unilateral lesion, irrespective of side of injury and presence or absence of seizures, leads to preservation of language skills at the expense of other functions, specifically visuospatial skills which may be 'crowded out' in the competition for neural space.

Taking into account our findings on young children with hemiplegia with those of other researchers who have studied older children, we need to acknowledge that successful reorganisation and preservation of function in the long term may be restricted to some but not all cognitive functions. It seems likely that higher order metalinguistic and educational skills, which develop in middle childhood, may not have such a good outcome in children with lateralised injury even when this has been sustained early in life, and possibly even after a promising start has been made in establishing early language and educational skills.

Implications for assessment and teaching

The research described above has important implications for the assessment and educational management of the child with hemiplegia. While all children with neurological impairment must be regarded as educationally vulnerable, it is likely that specific subgroups of children within the hemiplegic population may be especially 'at risk' for developing language and educational problems. These children in particular need to be targeted for increased and focused specialist learning support. On a cautionary note, however, referring to the findings from group-based predictor research as a basis for clinically identifying individual children at risk for learning is fraught with difficulties. A predictor variable that significantly predicts outcome in a group-based study may not on its own guarantee the reliable identification of individual children at risk. Specific cognitive factors always need to be evaluated in the context of the child's personal, family and schooling history as these provide powerful influences that can have far-reaching effects on a child's ultimate educational outcome.

Figure 13.1 depicts a proposed assessment framework for evaluating the cognitive abilities and educational attainments of children presenting with congenital hemiplegia. Specific tests are suggested which tap the primary cognitive and educational domains that should be assessed during the process of considering the special educational needs of the child with hemiplegia. Cases 13.1 and 13.2 describe assessment case histories of two children, both with congenital left-hemisphere injury, whose neuropsychological development was documented over a 2-year period. Reference is made to these case histories when considering the following general issues which relate to the assessment and management of the child with hemiplegia.

It is essential to take account of seizure status and also possibly the implications that type and dose of medication have for the child's functioning. Children with seizures appear to be at risk for generalised learning difficulties, while those with left-sided lesions might have the further disadvantage of additional specific language and educational problems which may make for a poorer long-term prognosis and which necessitate increased special needs provision.

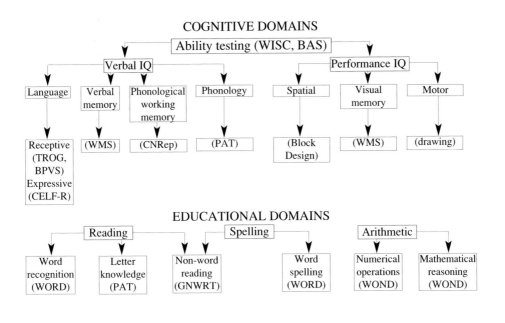

COGNITIVE DOMAINS

Ability testing (WISC, BAS)

Verbal IQ

Language — Receptive (TROG, BPVS) Expressive (CELF-R)

Verbal memory — (WMS)

Phonological working memory — (CNRep)

Phonology — (PAT)

Performance IQ

Spatial — (Block Design)

Visual memory — (WMS)

Motor — (drawing)

EDUCATIONAL DOMAINS

Reading

Word recognition (WORD)

Letter knowledge (PAT)

Non-word reading (GNWRT)

Spelling

Word spelling (WORD)

Arithmetic

Numerical operations (WOND)

Mathematical reasoning (WOND)

Key
WISC, Weschler Intelligence for Children (Weschler 1992)
BAS, British Abilities Scales (Elliot et al. 1983)
TROG, Test of Reception of Grammar (Bishop 1982)
BPVS, British Picture Vocabulary Scales (Dunn et al. 1992)
WMS, Weschler Memory Scales (Weschler and Stone 1945)
CNRep, Children's Test of Non-word Repetition (Gathercole and Baddeley 1997)
PAT, Phonological Abilities Test (Muter et al. 1997)
CELF-R, Clinical Evaluation of Language Eundamentals, Revised (Semel et al. 1987)
WORD, Weschler Objective Reading Dimensions (Rust et al. 1993)
WOND, Weschler Objective Numerical Dimensions (Rust 1996)
GNWRT, Graded Nonword Reading Test (Snowling et al. 1996)

Fig. 13.1. Proposed framework for assessing the cognitive and educational skills and needs of the child with hemiplegia

CASE 13.1

A neuropsychological profile of a child with left-hemisphere congenital injury without seizure complication

Patient 1 was first seen at age 5 years 7 months. He presented with a right-sided hemiplegia. A CT scan indicated the presence of a porencephalic cyst in the left-postcentral region, with atrophy of the adjacent frontal lobe. He had never experienced seizures.

At age 5 years 7 months, he obtained the following scores on the Wechsler Preschool and Primary Scale of Intelligence-Revised (WPPSI-R, Wechsler 1990):Verbal IQ = 110, Performance IQ = 95

Patient 1 is an able little boy. The size and direction of the Verbal–Performance discrepancy is consistent with that typically observed in children with congenital hemiplegia, irrespective of the side of injury.

Our patient had good concentration skills. On specific measures of language functioning (TROG,

BPVS and selected expressive measures from the CELF-R), he achieved at least age-appropriate scores. His verbal memory was well developed though he scored less well on measures of visual memory (children's version of the WMS). In respect of his phonological awareness, he was demonstrating the beginning of rhyming skill, and he could blend and segment syllables and phonemes within words (PAT). He was able to identify the sounds of all 26 letters of the alphabet.

At follow up 2 years later, patient 1 had retained his level and pattern of scoring on the Wechsler Scales (now the WISC-III, 1992). His visual memory, identified as an area of relative weakness 2 years earlier, appeared stronger. Our patient's phonological skills were developing very well indeed; he could detect and produce rhyme, he could blend and segment phonemes competently and he was making a very promising start in manipulating, specifically deleting, phonemes (PAT). His reading was age appropriate (WORD) and his spelling was within the normal range (WORD). However, he had markedly underdeveloped sequential decoding skill; he was unable to score on the test of non-word reading (GNWRT) which would place him at under the 6-year level for decoding ability.

CASE 13.2

A neuropsychological profile of a child with left-hemisphere congenital injury with seizure complication

This patient presented aged 4 years 10 months with a congenital right-hemiplegia. Her CT showed a left-hemisphere porencephalic cyst. She had one to two severe fits each year; she was treated with carbemazepine.

At age 4 years 10 months, our patient obtained the following scores on the WPPSI-R: Verbal IQ = 91, Performance IQ = 73.

The IQ scores are somewhat depressed relative to those of a child without hemiplegia and indeed relative to a non-seizure patient; the Verbal–Performance discrepancy favouring language over visually related skills is typical of the child with hemiplegia.

Our patient had poor attention skills at the initial assessment. Her receptive language skills (TROG and BPVS) were commensurate with her Verbal IQ, but aspects of her expressive language (CELF-R Formulated Sentences) were below the 3-year level. Her short-term memory (both verbal and visual) was very poor, and may have been markedly affected by her poor attention control. Her phonological sensitivity was restricted to simple syllable but not phoneme segmentation.

At follow up at age 6 years 10 months, our patient's IQ figures (WISC III) were maintained. Her short-term memory scores were relatively higher than at the original assessment, and concomitant with this was an observable improvement in her attention span and 'on-task' behaviour. She continued to register scores on selected expressive language tests that were below her ability level. Although, our patient's phonological skills had shown improvement (she could now blend and segment phonemes), they were not up to age expectation. Her letter knowledge (PAT) was incomplete (10 of 26 letters correctly identified), and she had only a minimum sight vocabulary in reading.

Our research has highlighted the need for comprehensive assessment of children's verbal and non-verbal skills, both in respect of gross function (which may be tapped by IQ tests) and specific and subtle language and educational deficits that may be particularly apparent in subjects with left-hemisphere insults and seizures. Our findings suggest that left-hemisphere injured children with seizures may be especially vulnerable to the development of specific learning difficulties in reading, spelling and mathematics. Recognising the heightened risk status of this subgroup of children with hemiplegia increases the likelihood of their learning difficulties being addressed at an early age before their educational problems become severe. Our patient in case 13.2 is a little girl who falls into this heightened at risk category. Her language and educational development need to be carefully monitored; she will very likely require access to literacy learning support and possibly also speech and language therapy.

The teaching of children with hemiplegia may involve different strategies and methods than those adopted for typicaly developing children. For instance, avoiding over-reliance on visually based learning strategies; or explicitly instructing intellectually capable children with left-hemisphere injury in phonology–reading connections, which appears to be an area of weakness for them. Our patient in case 13.1 is clearly having great difficulty in making the reading--phonology connection; adopting a teaching programme that emphasises linking sound segments to graphemic clusters will help to ensure that his developing word recognition vocabulary is securely underpinned in sound, thus preventing the danger of later reaching a plateau or having problems with spelling.

Recent research has highlighted the importance of recognising the individual child's cognitive strengths as well as weaknesses; consequently, there is a need to evaluate each child's relative strengths (in language, memory and so on) that might afford possible compensatory mechanisms. It is then possible for teachers to support, promote and reinforce these strengths and to teach compensatory strategies in order to improve the child's academic standards. In the verbally able child with hemiplegia, such as our patient in case 13.1, it may be profitable to encourage the child to take note of surrounding context in reading and to make use of semantic and syntactic cues when attacking unfamiliar words; in relying on good language abilities, the child is developing an effective compensator for the insecure phoneme–grapheme connections that make conventional decoding difficult.

Those involved in teaching children with hemiplegia need to be aware of the educational implications of their non-verbal deficits. Visuospatial weaknesses which are a feature of nearly all children with hemiplegia can make them vulnerable to problems in: acquiring mathematical concepts, such as understanding of fractions and Euclidean geometry; hand-writing; written presentation; and organisational skills in general; spatial aspects of the school curriculum such as interpreting maps and directions in geography; use of visual schema and diagrams in science. These pervasive and persisting non-verbal difficulties point to the importance of physical therapies and occupational therapy in helping children with hemiplegia develop improved visual, perceptual, spatial and fine motor coordination skills. There is evidence to show that the 'good' hand of children with hemiplegia is not as proficient as the preferred or even non-preferred hand of normal children in the execution of motor activities (Brown et al. 1989). In view of this, children with hemiplegia benefit from access to physical therapies that will help promote better coordination and pencil control, together with training in perceptual skills. They also require instruction and support from an early age in the use of computers and other technological aids.

Finally, given that many children with hemiplegia have normal intelligence, they can be expected to achieve academic standards that will enable them to take formal public examinations. Consequently, in line with the allowances afforded children with specific learning difficulties, it is necessary as part of their successful educational management to request allowances in examinations that include all or a combination of the following: extra time, use of word processors, concessions for handwriting and amanuensis.

ACKNOWLEDGEMENT

This chapter was prepared with the support of a grant from the Leverhulme Trust to the second author.

REFERENCES

Adams, M.J. (1990) *Beginning to Read: Thinking and Learning About Print.* Cambridge, MA: MIT Press.

Aram, D.M., Ekelman, B.L. (1986) Cognitive profiles of children with early onset of unilateral lesions. *Developmental Neuropsychology,* **2,** 155–172.

—— (1988) Scholastic aptitude and achievement among children with unilateral brain lesions. *Neuropsychologia,* **26,** 903–916.

—— Whitaker, H.A. (1986) Spoken syntax in children with acquired unilateral hemisphere lesions. *Brain and Language,* **27,** 75–100.

——— (1987) Lexical retrieval in left- and right-brain lesioned children. *Brain and Language,* **31,** 61–89.

— Eisele, J.A. (1994) Intellectual stability in children with unilateral brain lesions. *Neuropsychologia,* **28,** 85–95.

Banich, M.T., Levine, S.C., Kim, H., Huttenlocher, P. (1990) The effects of developmental factors on IQ in hemiplegic children. *Neuropsychologia,* **28,** 35–47.

Bates, E. (1992) Language development. *Current Opinion in Neurobiology,* **2,** 180–185.

— Vicari, S., Trauner, D. (1999) Neural mediation of language development: perspectives from lesion studies of infants and children. *In:* Tager-Flusberg, H. (Ed.). *Neurodevelopmental Disorders:* Cambridge, MA: MIT Press. p. 533–581.

Bishop, D.V.M. (1982) *Test of Reception of Grammar, TROG.* Available from D. Bishop, Dept of Experimental Psychology, University of Oxford, South Parks Road, Oxford OX1 3UD, UK.

— (1983) Linguistic impairment after hemidecortication for infantile hemiplegia? A reappraisal. *Quarterly Journal of Experimental Psychology,* **35,** 199–207.

— (1988) Can the right hemisphere mediate language as well as the left? A critical review of recent research. *Cognitive Neuropsychology,* **5,** 353–367.

Carlsson, G., Hugdahl, K., Uvebrant, P., Wiklund, L-M., Von Wendt, L. (1992) Pathological left-handedness revisited: Dichotic listening in children with left versus right hemiplegia. *Neuropsychologia,* **30,** 471–481.

— Uvebrant, P., Hugdahl, K., Arvidsson, J., Wiklund, L-M., Von Wendt, L. (1994) Verbal and non-verbal function of children with right versus left hemiplegic cerebral palsy of pre- and peri-natal origin. *Developmental Medicine and Child Neurology,* **36,** 503–512.

Dorman, C. (1987) Verbal, perceptual and intellectual factors associated with reading achievement in adolescents with cerebral palsy. *Perceptual and Motor Skills,* **64,** 671–678.

Dunn, L.N., Dunn, L.M., Whetton, C. (1982) *British Picture Vocabulary Scale.* Windsor, UK: NFER-Nelson.

Eisele, J., Aram, D. (1994) Comprehension and imitation of syntax following early hemisphere damage. *Brain and Language,* **46,** 212–231.

Elliott, C.D., Murray D.J., Pearson, L.S. (1983) *British Ability Scales.* Windsor, UK: NFER-Nelson.

Frampton, I., Yude, C., Goodman, R. (1998) Learning problems in children with hemiplegia. *British Journal of Educational Psychology,* **68,** 39–51.

Gathercole, S., Baddeley, A. (1997) *Children's Test of Nonword Repetition (CNRep).* London: Psychological Corporation, Harcourt-Brace.

Goldman, P.S. (1974) An alternative to developmental plasticity: heterology of CNS structures in infants and adults. *In:* Stein D. G., Rosen J.J., Butters N (Eds). *Plasticity and Recovery of Function in the Central Nervous System.* New York: Academic Press.

Goodman, R., Yude, C. (1996) IQ and its predictors in childhood hemiplegia. *Developmental Medicine and Child Neurology,* **38,** 881–890.

Goswami, U., Bryant, P. (1990) *Phonological Skills and Learning to Read.* London: Erlbaum.

Haskell, S.H. (1966) *Arithmetical Disabilities in Cerebral Palsied Children.* Springfield, IL: Charles Thomas.

Hebb, D.O. (1942) The effect of early and late brain injury upon test scores, and the nature of normal adult intelligence. *Proceedings of the American Philosophical Society,* **85,** 275–292.

Hiscock, M., Decter, M.H. (1988) Dichotic listening in children. *In:* Hugdahl, K. (Ed.) *Handbook of Dichotic Listening: Theory, Methods and Research.* 431–473. Chichester, UK: John Wiley and Sons.

Hulme, C., Snowling, M. (1992) Deficits in output phonology: An explanation for reading failure. *Cognitive Neuropsychology,* **9,** 47–72.

Isaacs, E., Christie, D., Vargha-Khadem, F., Mishkin, M. (1996) Effects of hemispheric side of injury, age at injury and presence of seizure disorder on functional ear and hand asymmetries in hemiplegic children. *Neuropsychologia, 34*, 127–137.

Karmiloff-Smith, A. (1992) *Beyond Modularity: A Developmental Perspective on Cognitive Science*. Cambridge, MA: Bradford.

Kimura, D. (1961) Cerebral dominance and the perception of verbal stimuli. *Canadian Journal of Psychology, 15*, 166–171.

Lenneberg, E.H. (1967) *Biological Foundations of Language*. New York: Wiley.

Levine, S.C., Huttenlocher, P.R., Banich, M.T., Duda, E. (1987) Factors affecting cognitive functioning in hemiplegic children. *Developmental Medicine and Child Neurology, 29*, 27–35.

McCarthy, R.A., Warrington, E.K. (1990) Cognitive neuropsychology: A clinical introduction. San Diego, CA: Academic Press.

Muter, V.A. (1994) *Phonology and Learning to Read in Normal and Hemiplegic Children*. University of London PhD thesis.

— Hulme, C., Snowling, M. (1997) *Phonological Abilities Test (PAT)*. London: Psychological Corporation, Harcourt-Brace.

— Taylor, S., Vargha-Khadem, F. (1997) A longitudinal study of early intellectual development in hemiplegic children. *Neuropsychologia, 35*, 289–298.

— Snowling, M. (1998) Concurrent and longitudinal predictors of reading: The role of metalinguistic and short-term memory skills. *Reading Research Quarterly, 33*, 320–335.

Plunkett, K., Karmiloff-Smith, A., Bates, E., Elman, J.L., Johnson, M. (1997) Connectionism and developmental psychology. *Journal of Child Psychology and Psychiatry, 38*, 53–80.

Rack, J., Snowling. M., Olson, R. (1992) The nonword reading deficit in developmental dyslexia. *Reading Research Quarterly, 27*, 29–53.

Rankin, J.M., Aram, D.M., Horowitz, S.J. (1981) Language ability in right and left hemiplegic children. *Brain and Language, 14*, 292–306.

Rasmussen, T., Milner, B. (1977) The role of early left-brain injury in determining lateralisation of cerebral speech functions. *Annals of the New York Academy of Sciences, 299*, 355–369.

Reilly, J., Bates, E., Marchman, V. (1998) Narrative discourse in children with early focal brain injury. *In:* Dennis M, (Ed.). *Brain and Language - Discourse in Children with Anomalous Brain Development or Acquired Brain Injury, 61*, 335–375.

Rust, J., Golombok, S., Trickey, G. (1993) *Wechsler Objective Reading Dimensions*. London: Psychological Corporation, Harcourt-Brace.

— (1996) *Wechsler Objective Numerical Dimensions*. London: Psychological Corporation, Harcourt-Brace.

Satz, P., Strauss, E., Whitaker, H. (1990) The ontogeny of hemispheric specialisation: Some old hypotheses revisited. *Brain and Language, 38*, 596–614.

Semel, E., Wiig, E.H., Secord, W. (1987) *Clinical Evaluation of Language Fundamentals -Revised (CELF-R)*. London: Psychological Corporation, Harcourt-Brace.

Shallice, T. (1988) Phonological agraphia and the lexical route of writing. *Brain, 104*, 413–429.

Snowling, M., Stothard, S., MacLean, J. (1996) *Graded Nonword Reading Test*. Bury St Edmunds, UK: Thames Valley.

Temple, C.M. (1997) Cognitive neuropsychology and its application to children. *Journal of Child Psychology and Psychiatry, 38*, 27-52.

Teuber, H-L. (1975) Recovery of function after brain injury in man. *In:* Porter, R., Fitzsimmons, D. W. (Eds.). *Outcome of Severe Damage to the Central Nervous System. CIBA Foundation Symposium* 34. 159–190. Elsevier: Amsterdam.

Thal, D., Bates, E., Goodman, J., Jahn-Samilo, J. (1997) Continuity of language abilities in late- and early-talking toddlers. *In:* Thal D., Reilly, J. (Eds.). Special issue on Origins of Communication Disorders, *Developmental Neuropsychology, 13*, 239–273.

Vargha-Khadem, F. (1993) Congenital vs acquired insult of the cerebral hemispheres: Neuropsychological perspectives. *Educational and Child Psychology,* (Special Issue: The Brain and Behaviour: Organic Influences on the Behaviour of Children. Besag F. M. C., Williams R. T. [Guest Eds]). *10*, 12–16.

— Isaacs, E., Van Der Werf, S., Robb, S., Wilson, J. (1992) Development of intelligence and memory in children with hemiplegic cerebral palsy. *Brain, 115*, 315–329.

—— Muter, V. (1994) A review of cognitive outcome after unilateral lesions sustained during childhood. *Journal of Child Neurology, 9*, 2S67–2S73.

— Mishkin, M. (1997) Speech and language outcome after hemispherectomy in childhood. *In:* Tuxhorn, I.,. Holthausen, H., Boenigk H. E. (Eds.). *Paediatric Epileptic Syndromes and Their Surgical Treatment.* London: J. Libbey. p 774–784.

Wechsler, D. (1942) *Wechsler Memory Scales.* San Antonio, TX: Psychological Corporation. Adaptation for children after Milner, B. (1975) Psychological aspects of focal epilepsy and its neurosurgical management. *Advances in Neurology,* **8,** 299–321.

—(1963) *Wechsler Pre-school and Primary Scale of Intelligence .* London: Psychological Corporation, Harcourt Brace.

— (1976) *Wechsler Intelligence Scale for Children - Revised* (WISC-R). London: Psychological Corporation, Harcourt Brace.

—(1990) *Wechsler Pre-school and Primary Scale of Intelligence-(Revised).* London: Psychological Corporation, Harcourt Brace.

— (1992) *Wechsler Intelligence Scale for Children - III* (WISC-III). London: Psychological Corporation, Harcourt Brace.

Woodcock, R. W., Johnson, M. D. (1977) *The Woodcock-Johnson Psycho-educational Battery.* Hingham, MA: Teaching Resources.

14
SUPPORTING PARENTS OF CHILDREN WITH HEMIPLEGIA

Carole Yude

The Children Act (1989) placed a duty on local authorities to inform parents of children diagnosed with a disabling or medical condition about any voluntary organisations which could offer them support. In the UK, the organisation *Contact a Family*, publishes a directory which lists over 200 such groups supporting around 800 conditions, ranging from umbrella organisations to small groups of perhaps six or seven families whose children have rare disorders. Many of the well-known national voluntary organisations began their lives as small groups of parents coming together for mutual support, while others were initiated through specialist clinics for specific disorders. Hemi-Help is one of the few parent support groups to have started directly through a research project.

The background

In compiling a research register of families whose children have a specific condition and entering into a research partnership with them, a responsibility is placed on the researchers to both support and inform those families. During the first 3 years (1989 to 1991) of an epidemiological study to investigate the causes and consequences of childhood hemiplegia, the London Hemiplegia Register (LHR) recruited 463 families whose children were aged 0 to 16 years. One-hundred and forty-nine of these families with children aged between 6 and 10 years took part in a more intensive phase of the study including semistructured parent interviews and neuropsychological assessment. From the outset the researchers set out to inform parents and children about the progress of the LHR research, and that of others in the field, through a quarterly newsletter. Hemi-Help was initiated by the researchers and a small group of parents in the third year of the study and obtained charity status in the following year. Families on the research register were invited to join Hemi-Help and 300 (66%) became members. Hemi-Help is now a national organisation currently standing at around 1700 families and professionals. Its aims and objectives are 'to provide information and support to children with hemiplegia and their families' and to raise awareness of the condition among both professionals and the public.

Why start a group specifically for hemiplegia?

Hemiplegia is generally classified as a form of cerebral palsy (CP), though not all clinicians would agree with this definition. The question arises as to why a group specifically supporting children with hemiplegia was started when a national organisation supporting people with CP was already in existence? The simple answer was need and a direct response to parents wishes.

In the first 3 years of the LHR study, parents were asked, through a postal questionnaire, whether they were, or had ever been, members of a parent support group, or voluntary organisation. At that time, of the 463 families surveyed, only 4% were currently members of any support group and 9% were formerly members. During the interview stage of the study, parents were asked why they did not belong to a parent support group, or if they had been members in the past, why they had left.

Most of the dissatisfaction was inextricably linked to information given to them about hemiplegia at the time of diagnosis. Hemiplegia is sometimes categorised as CP, albeit a mild form, and sometimes in more general terms as a motor disorder. Thus parents who had initially joined the larger organisations reported that they had felt marginalised in groups which supported children with more severe physical disabilities given the diversity of the cerebral palsies. Even when other conditions associated with hemiplegia, for example, epilepsy and specific learning or more global learning difficulties became apparent parents mentioned that they were uncertain which of the major parent support organisations was the most appropriate. Yet by far the most frequent answer to the question of why parents felt unsupported by the current provision was because they had been told at an early stage that they were lucky that their child had a mild condition like hemiplegia. This made them feel that their child did not qualify as having special needs and as a consequence they, as a family, did not require extra support.

Despite their dissatisfaction with existing services, parents were all too aware that they did need support from other parents in the same situation and more importantly they needed information about education. Educational provision for children with special needs had been in a perpetual state of change since the 1981 Education Act established the right of such children to equal access to education and to their increasing integration in mainstream schools. Further modifications only added to the confusion of parents seeking adequate support for their children. By the third year of the LHR study parents on the research register were reporting that the quarterly newsletter was a lifeline offering information about hemiplegia directly from the research and reassurance that other parents were experiencing similar problems with their child. The correspondence increased with each issue. The predominating concerns were as might have been expected – early physical and cognitive development, education, therapy, behavioural management and equipment. Clearly parents needed a forum to share their concerns, especially the psychological problems they were encountering in their children as they grew up. The continuation of this newsletter, the doubling of the mailing list from both families who were not involved in the research study and from interested professionals and the uncertainty of continuing research funds were all instrumental in the invitation to parents to form a support group, and so Hemi-Help was born.

What form should a parent support group take?

Fundamental to all models of working with families is an understanding of the way in which parents adjust to the recognition that the child they expected to develop in the normal way has significant long-term problems. This can be most easily explained within a stages analysis and has been expressed by Hornby (1995) as follows:

Shock → denial → anger → sadness → detachment → reorganisation → acceptance.

Parents progress along this continuum, slipping in and out of stages, and frequently backwards from time to time – particularly when life events remind them of what might have been. As a general principle, parents may need to reach the stage of reorganisation before they are ready to join a professionally managed support group because membership implies public acknowledgement of their child's disability, although they may obtain support from a smaller less focused parent-led group in the interim. A call to a helpline or a request for literature is often the first approach made to an organisation simply because it requires neither disclosure nor commitment from the enquirer. For other parents, just knowing that a group exists, should they need it, may be sufficient: meeting other parents can sometimes be helpful and sometimes not. Some understanding of the way that parents adjust to their child's disability, whether it is explained within a stages analysis or any other psychological process, is required when planning the model of parental support to be offered.

Models of parent support

Parent support groups initiated and run by professionals are likely to be multidisability groups, located in a local clinic, hospital, or special-school setting. All of these provide parents with a forum to exchange information, discuss problems, share feelings, offer support and also arrive at solutions with some professional help. As such, they could, according Tavormina's (1974) definition, be described as reflective or introspective groups focused on personal issues. Professionals may also make use of these groups as a research resource to formulate research questions, monitor intervention programmes or shifts in coping strategies and so on. Other groups have been established to train parents in the management of their children's problem behaviours (Webster-Stratton and Herbert 1994).

The larger voluntary organisations provide more extensive information facilities, assessment facilities and advocacy. Although these larger organisations have a great deal to offer, some parents have described them as helpful when seeking specific information or assessment services, but impersonal when more individually focused support is needed. Smaller groups offer parents the opportunity to get together for mutual support, leading to better personal coping strategies and personal growth. As Hornby (1995) points out the larger the group, the greater the loss of therapeutic factors. Parents have a great deal to gain from support groups, whether they are 'reflective or introspective' as described above or focused on behavioural management as in the Webster-Stratton and Herbert (1994) model where parents gain knowledge, control and learn effective coping skills. However, combining the aspects of both approaches may well prove to have the best outcome for parents who are dealing with a multiplicity of problems, not least of which is their own adjustment to their child.

Whether Hemi-Help fits into any one model of parental support is by no means clear-cut. Basically it is a parent-to-parent group in an informal partnership with a research project and can perhaps be described as a model led by parents with advice from professionals. From its inception, Hemi-Help decided not to become affiliated to a larger organisation, although a considerable amount of help was received from the development officers of such an organisation during the early stages. Parent-to-parent groups generally provide training in basic counselling or listening skills for those operating the information- or helpline. Although Hemi-Help does not act as a linking organisation, in some circumstances parents can be put in touch with another parent, close either in terms of geography or whose child has similar problems. Parent-to-parent support given by trained parent volunteers on the telephone also provides a unique perspective helpful to parents of newly diagnosed children which only people who have been through a similar experience can offer. The issues that predominated in the early days of the LHR newsletter correspondence continue to be paramount; namely, early development – both physical and cognitive, education, therapy, behavioural management and equipment. As the children of the original members reach adulthood, parental concerns about further education, work, driving, independence, marriage and children are becoming more important.

Are parent support groups useful and effective?

There is very little formal evaluation of the effectiveness of parent groups in the literature, although there is considerable anecdotal evidence to endorse their value. Indeed there is a view that voluntary organisations are a determining factor in how well families cope (Hornby 1995). However, there has been a shift from the early 1980s when Holland and Hattersley reported that their group supporting parents of children with learning disabilities was primarily a clinical service. Current models involve more collaborative parent–professional partnerships where there is a mutual acknowledgement of individual expertise and a sharing of knowledge and skills to benefit the family and the child (Cunningham and Davis 1985, Webster-Stratton and Herbert 1994, Hornby 1995). In practical terms, Hemi-Help is evaluated every day by its members. If parents' needs were unmet, they would simply cease to be members. Although Hemi-Help continually monitors its progress through feedback from its members, the formal evaluative process can be time consuming, costly and painful (De'Ath 1983).

Hemi-Help is based on various models and itself acts as a model for other smaller parent-led groups. Due to the involvement of parents, Hemi-Help has incorporated some of the elements of Egan's model of the 'skilled helper' (Egan 1981) into its training – that is to be non-directive, to empower parents and to help them develop their problem-solving skills. Hemi-Help does not act as an advocate for parents but endeavours to help parents to become advocates for their own children in order to get the best possible services for them. Hemi-Help brings together parents to share common concerns through the newsletter and parent workshops, enabling them to feel reassured and supported by contact with others in the same situations with similar goals. In order to be effective, Hemi-Help maintains a flexible, loosely structured framework which is open to the needs of its members. Although Hemi-Help's management committee is primarily parent led, it is able to tap into areas of professional expertise through its links with the LHR research study.

As an organisation Hemi-Help decided, after much discussion, that it would not jump on the band wagon of the latest miracle solution to a specific problem and chose on two counts never to endorse a specific treatment, a particular hospital, clinic or school. First, because Hemi-Help is a small organisation with limited resources and would find it difficult to evaluate the various treatments or centres and second, the organisation would be open to litigation from dissatisfied parents if their endorsement proved to be ill founded. However, Hemi-Help does, on request, put parents in touch with each other so that they can offer individual advice on a parent-to-parent basis.

What can Hemi-Help offer its members?

Hemi-Help produces a quarterly newsletter in which parents can be informed about changes in educational legislation and current advances in research. Parents also use the newsletter to share experiences and request and exchange information.

The information or helpline which primarily affords parents the opportunity to talk to a trained volunteer, can also offer help with aids, equipment and other useful organisations from a database of information about hemiplegia and its associated conditions.

Hemi-Help's literature is based on its own area of expertise and is directed specifically at the difficulties associated with hemiplegia. A *What is Hemiplegia?* leaflet was initially developed in response to parents' requests for a description of hemiplegia in plain English suitable for grandparents and the extended family. Now in its second edition it has become the first information leaflet to be offered to the parents of a newly diagnosed child. Since the majority of children with hemiplegia attend mainstream schools, Hemi-Help's two different *Guidelines for Teachers* have been written for teachers of 5 to 11 year olds and 12 to 18 year olds respectively.

Don't Give Up; Growing Up with Hemiplegia, a professional video for younger children made with the help of adolescents has been most successful in helping young people with hemiplegia to see that they are not alone as they tackle problems from teasing to shoe-lace tying, take part in and succeed at sports and other leisure activities, and talk about their lives and hopes for the future. Other fact sheets supply information on individual topics and resources.

Regular parent workshops are held where parents can meet in informal circumstances to hear about recent research into hemiplegia, current treatments and educational matters. A professionally managed creche allows parents the freedom to participate in the workshops without their child. It also gives the children with hemiplegia and their siblings the chance to meet and play together. Many children with hemiplegia attending mainstream schools, have never met another child like themselves and so the creche is a particularly valuable resource for covert comparisons and mutual understanding.

Fun and activity days are also a regular fixture in the Hemi-Help year. To date, Hemi-Help has organised sports days, sailing events and music workshops where children with hemiplegia, their siblings and friends, can participate, with expert coaching, in many activities they might not otherwise attempt.

Future projects include a leaflet specifically aimed at preschool children, an interactive CD-Rom to be used as a training and information resource for professionals and a web site.

Is Hemi-Help meeting the needs of the membership?

Five years after its inception, and with 1000 members at that time, Hemi-Help undertook a membership survey – with some interesting results. Approximately a third of the membership

TABLE 14.1
Responses to Hemi-Help questionnaire rating 10 activities in order of priority

	Parents	*Professionals*
1	Newsletter	Newsletter
2	Helpline	Information on current research
3	Sympathetic ear for newly disgnosed families	Helpline
4	User-friendly leaflets and information about hemiplegia	User-friendly leaflets and information about hemiplegia
5	Information on current research	Information on resources and equipment
6	Parent workshops	
7	Information on resources and equipment	
8	Video	
9	Children's activity days	
10	Linking parents with each other	

returned their questionnaires and the results were divided into two groups for analysis – parents and professionals. The focus of the survey was to find out: what Hemi-Help did best; how well Hemi-Help was doing it; and how to increase Hemi-Help's revenue in order to continue its activities

All respondents, both parents and professionals, were asked to rate the 10 activities listed in order of priority (Table 14.1). As might have been expected, parents, who rated all 10 services, use Hemi-Help's services somewhat differently to professionals who rated only five of the services that Hemi-Help offers. Parents reported that:

• the newsletter was a lifeline

• the leaflets for teachers gave them confidence to explain the problems and demand support

• the helpline was invaluable – whether seeking specific information or just someone to talk to

• the fun/activity days allowed children with hemiplegia to attempt sports and activities that as parents they had discounted owing to the nature of their child's disability.

• the workshops brought parents together (as also evidenced by the fact that the tea breaks are getting longer and the presentations much shorter – there is obviously a need to share experiences).

• professionals working with children with hemiplegia reported that Hemi-Help was a valuable resource.

Funding a parent support group

Hemi-Help began with various small start-up grants and it was decided from the outset not to levy a membership fee in order that no family should be precluded from becoming a member. Hemi-Help has been fortunate in its fund-raising activities and still has no membership fee nor does it charge for literature, children's activity days, or parent workshops and the professional creche it provides there. Until 1998 when the first paid worker was appointed, Hemi-Help had been run entirely by volunteers.

What does the membership want from Hemi-Help?

The results of the survey demonstrated clearly what the membership wants from Hemi-Help in concrete terms. Yet when talking to parents at workshops and on the helpline what emerges as the most important factor is not so much what is produced in terms of services but just knowing that Hemi-Help is there. To use the stages analysis once more, parents have varying needs depending on where they are on the continuum. An analysis of the database indicates that parents seek information from parent-support groups when their child is first diagnosed, although they do not necessarily join at this time, usually becoming members around the time of preschool or school entry. In middle childhood most children and families are getting on with their lives, with the next peak of involvement around the time of secondary-school transfer. As yet Hemi-Help has had little success in starting a group for young adults with hemiplegia – perhaps because they too are getting on with their lives and do not want to be identified with a disability group.

For some parents just receiving the newsletter may be sufficient. Travelling 100 miles to a parent workshop and meeting other parents may be important for others. Some may prefer a one-to-one link with another parent or perhaps a chat to someone on the helpline in a moment of despair. What is certain is that no one parent support group can meet the needs of all the membership all the time, but they need to be there for the times when they can.

REFERENCES

Children Act (1989) Schedule II, part 1, para 1(2). London: HMSO.

Cunningham, C., Davis, H. (1985) *Working with Parents: Frameworks for Collaboration.* Open University Press.

De'Ath, E. (1983) *Evaluating Parents' Groups.* National Children's Bureau.

Education Act (1981) Chap 60, section 2(2). London: Department for Education for England and Wales.

Egan, G. (1981) *The Skilled Helper.* Monterey, CA: Brooks/Cole.

Holland, J., Hattersley, J. (1980) Parent support groups for the families of mentally handicapped children. *Child, Care and Development,* **6**, 165–173

Hornby, G. (1995) *Working with Parents of Children with Special Needs.* London: Cassell

Tavormina, J. B. (1974) Basic models of parent counselling: A critical review. *Psychological Bulletin,* **81**, 827–835.

Webster-Stratton, C., Herbert, M. (1994) *Troubled Families, Problem Children. Working with Parents: A Collaborative Process.* Chichester: John Wiley.

USEFUL ORGANISATIONS

Contact a Family, 100 Tottenham Court Road London W1P OHA.
Tel: 020 73833555   Fax: 020 73830259
Hemi-Help, Bedford House, 215 Balham High Road, London SW17 7BQ.
Tel: 020 86723179   Fax: 020 87670319   www.hemihelp.org.uk
SCOPE, 6 Market Road, London N7 9PW
Tel: 020 76197100   Fax: 020 76197399

15
A COMMUNITY-LEVEL SERVICE FOR CHILDREN WITH CONGENITAL HEMPLEGIA

Brian Neville

This chapter assumes that families have the right to expect a locally based community disability service through which the clinical team can:
• identify impairments and disabilities
• supply specific treatments
• give advice on management issues
• access specialist services where necessary and coordinate these within a community-based service
• liaise with education, social and community services
• provide linkage with appropriate adult services.

Such a service should attempt to find solutions for specific problems and to meet defined goals both for individuals and for the whole service. This requires individual management plans for each child, guidelines for problem solving and the management of specific impairments, and a strategic-planning level of management. The latter aspect of management develops the service in response to data that emerge from each multidisciplinary team using their current guidelines. It has to assess the performance of the service against its own goals, to respond to medical advances; to listen to parents and people with disabling conditions, and to decide on the use of resources. Issues that need to be addressed within strategic planning include:
• the balance between locally based services and the use of more specialised services at greater distance from people's homes
• the balance between high-quality individual services and poor coverage of the population
• a balance of service components between those which arise from the strengths and inclination of the staff and those which are put forward by the client group
• the priority of medical interventions compared with community support and education.

A local disability service is likely to be tested by the child with hemiplegia due to the wide range of problems these children experience. Reading this book, it is clear that the service has to be comprehensive, covering all domains of disability. The notion that children with the cerebral palsies should be primarily managed by services for physical disabilities is nonsense and calls into question the setting up of pure cerebral palsy services in various parts of the world. The designation 'orthopaedically handicapped', used widely in India for example, for people with physical disability, is plainly either wrong or often an unfortunately accurate description of the predicament of people with hemiplegia faced with isolated surgical 'expertise'.

In some parts of the world community-based services for those with a disability are not provided and, therefore, the family has to attempt to coordinate their child's care through office- and hospital-based practice. This cannot be regarded as appropriate yet it is interesting how this is the case in a number of affluent countries. Community-based services would be cheaper as well as more likely to provide better coverage of the population and to involve community agencies both to integrate services and also people with disabilities within the community (McConachie and Zinkin 1995).

Most child development services would not claim to have a specific service for children with hemiplegia. At best this could mean that all their needs are catered for whatever the medical diagnosis and at worst that the children who mostly walk and talk have their psychosocial needs ignored unless they come into contact with an epilepsy service which may provide such care. The chances of the epilepsy services being integrated into a disability service are, however, quite small. The discrepancies between what is offered, the level of need as perceived by the support group Hemi-Help (see preceding chapter), and the medical evidence which this book has collated make a very strong case for the early ascertainment of children with hemiplegia. This would be of particular value in an effort to help with behaviour problems at an early stage if necessary. How this is accomplished within a programme which is trying to provide for the needs of all children with disabilities is for a local team to decide with the help of its parent support groups. The strongest message for child development services over the past 10 to 20 years has been the growing power and influence of parent support groups with whom medical professionals must develop a trusting working relationship. Using this partnership, many of the needs of families can be taken out of the medical arena and met by the resources of their support groups, using medical professionals where necessary. Tensions will develop sometimes as individual parents seek to use specific therapies, non-traditional therapies or as they look for a particular level of support. The better the working relationship between parents and professionals the easier it should be to engage in a discussion of scientific evidence and practical issues so that priorities can be developed jointly. The production of national and international guidelines for services' provision is an achievable aim. The European Academy of Childhood Disability has recently produced a useful start in this process in a review of how services are provided in Europe (EACD 1997).

Most families appreciate systems of management in which a professional takes a key-worker role for the family throughout their management. Ideally this is someone with whom they have shared the early painful experiences of diagnosis and who can help in deciding on priorities. This may be crucial when an enthusiastic therapist wants a great deal of effort to be put into encouraging function in a hand with dense sensory and motor deficit, or exercises to prevent scoliosis in early life, or orthotic treatment and surgery for equinus in a child with autistic features who is terrified of the medical treatment. Each of these three approaches are both futile and potentially harmful activities but they sometimes happen and in situations in which the relative merits and disadvantages are more difficult to assess. This prioritising approach must extend to intervention by specialist services which must coordinate their input with that of the local team. This relationship becomes difficult if it seems to the specialist unit that the community team is making a clinical mistake. The best method of dealing with these situations is if the specialist unit offers consultations as part of the service at community level, and that the two services develop guidelines jointly for the management of common conditions. It is also important that neonatal units ensure that babies at high risk of disability are seen early by the appropriate child development team early. Legitimate professional interest in outcome can be achieved by integrating neonatal follow up into community disability services.

Before significant interventions occur the family and child, if developmentally feasible, should be given an opportunity to express their views on what they are hoping for and discuss with medical professionals what can be achieved. These should be written down and form the basis for the decision on proceedings and for future audit. This has proved a simple but effective tool in epilepsy surgery (Taylor et al. 1997).

Meeting the specific medical needs of children with hemiplegia must include the availability of, but not necessarily the use of, physiotherapy, occupational therapy, orthotic and orthopaedic surgery. Surgery for the cerebral palsies is a specialist area and with the possibility of a range of antispasticity treatments should be performed by people with specialist training and competence in the field who manage such problems within a multidisciplinary team.

The psychiatric and social issues have been discussed in detail in this book, but how is help to be delivered? These problems include attention deficit, hyperactivity, autistic features, depression, and difficulties of social adjustment and peer-group relationships. They are common and they are shared with many other children with disabilities of cerebral origin. Some of the factors involved in the provision, or lack of it, of behavioural services for children with disabilities are:
• they have very large numbers of children to deal with, for example, a UK local area service for a total population of 200 000 will have hundreds of such children
• very few child psychiatrists and other mental health professionals are fully integrated into childhood disability teams, or have the requisite training in paediatric disability.
• the usual time requirements for mental health consultations make their routine involvement impossible.
• the practical approach to psychiatric problems has to be to use the personnel of the child development team to build behavioural management within their whole approach.

Thus the leader of behavioural services should be within the disability team and deploy the strengths of parents, statutory (particularly nursing) staff and voluntary workers and education and social services. Meeting the cognitive needs of children with hemiplegia should be coordinated with the behavioural services and to achieve this it is imperative that educational psychology is also integrated with the disability team, i.e. that educational and medical services are integrated.

For inexplicable reasons epilepsy services are not usually integrated into disability services despite the very high rate of additional impairments, particularly cognitive and behavioural, in children with intractable epilepsy. However, in children with congenital hemiplegia and epilepsy such integrated care is essential. The early selection of some children for assessment for surgical treatment and the need to balance seizure relief with both positive and negative behavioural effects of treatment are powerful reasons for early neurological input. Following any surgery there is a need for rehabilitation.

Ophthalmic and audiological services should be available within the same integrated service. This account of disability services points to the need for the efficient deployment of services which have usually been separately developed and have not always been put together into a unified programme. There are more radical approaches to community-based care which are only referred to briefly. These include community-based rehabilitation programmes which put all resources under the control of community agencies. Many different approaches have been used in developing and developed countries (McConachie and Zinkin 1995) but some principles could be used more widely, for example, that people with disabilities and their families should be brought into the development and management of services as equal partners; that all clinical interventions (and non-clinical for that matter) should come under the same community scrutiny whether or not they are what would normally be regarded as part of acute or disability neurology.

The ways that families cope when their eagerly awaited child is discovered to have an impairment have been discussed elsewhere in detail as have the need for professionals to be trained in the process of revealing problems and the methods of helping families to use the resources available to them (McCarthy 1992). The extra dimensions in congenital hemiplegia are the frequent difficulties with early diagnosis and perhaps more the process of slow revelation of the extent of the disability complex with time so that the family face the possibility of several life events not just one. The prediction that the use of an MRI-derived pathological diagnosis in the cerebral palsies would allow better prediction of the expected phenotype is now a realistic possibility. Separating the outcome of pure white-matter involvement from extensive cortical grey-matter damage (with a much higher rate of cognitive, behavioural and seizure impairments) could be helpful and be part of a process by which the cerebral palsies are classified and managed to a considerable extent by their pathology rather than the anatomical distribution of their impairments.

REFERENCES

European Academy of Childhood Disability (1997) Services for childhood disability in Europe. *Developmental Medicine and Child Neurology* **39: (Suppl. 76).**
McCarthy, G. (1992) *Physical Disability in Childhood: An Interdisciplinary Approach to Management.* Edinburgh: Churchill Livingstone.
McConachie, H., Zinkin, P. (Eds) (1995) *Disabled Children and Developing Countries. Clinics in Developmental Medicine No. 136.* London: Mac Keith Press.
Taylor, D.C., Neville, B.G.R., Cross, J.H. (1997) New measures of outcome needed for the surgical treatment of epilepsy. *Epilepsia* **38:** 625–630. (Editorial).

INDEX

(Page numbers in *italics* refer to figures/tables.)

A

abduction orthosis, 98
activity anticipation, 118
adductor longus, surgical division, 106
adductor policis muscle, 127
adulthood, 79
adults, outcome, 177
aetiology of congenital hemiplegia, 2–4
aggression, 169, 170
agyria, 18–19, 28
Aicardi syndrome, X-linked 20
alcohol injection, 144
ankle
  clonus, 67, 124–125
  dorsiflexion, 56
  double-bump pattern, *83*, 84
  equinus deformity, 69, 138–139
  plantarflexion, 67
  plantarflexor abnormal stance phase function,
      103–104
  plantarflexor/dorsiflexor imbalance, 103
  sagittal plane motion, 83, *85*
  video recordings, 94
ankle–foot orthosis (AFO), 68, 78–79, 93, 98
  ankle plantarflexor abnormal stance phase function,
      103–104
  valgus deformity, 164
  young children, 165
anorexia nervosa, 171
anticonvulsants, 154
antiphospholipid antibodies, 44
antisocial behaviour, 170
anxiety
  disorders, 169, 171
  parents, 173
  treatmen, 176
Apgar scores, 10
arm
  flexion, 115
  manipulative skill failure, 125
  movement difficulties, 55
  parachute response, 125, *126*
  posture, 139
  shortening, 58
  swinging, 119, 139
  windmill movement, 127
artificial limbs, 123

asphyxia in reflex hemisyndrome, 124
aspirin, prophylactic, 158
assessment of children, 188, 190–191
astrocytes, atypical, 20–21
asymmetry of function, 75
ataxia, 119
athetoid movements, 58
athetosis, 119
attachment figures, 169
attention deficit, 167–168
audiological services, 205
auditory perceptual deficiencies, central, 60
autism/autistic features, 170–171
autistic problems, 177
autonomic nervous system, 142
autosomal dominant trait, 2
awareness of affected side, 76

B

Babinski sign, 6
  positive, 57, 58
baclofen, intrathecal, 132, 137
  abnormal postures, 146
  plasticity, 141
baclofen, oral, 144
balloon cells, 20
basal ganglia, 119
behavioural problems, 166–167, 169–170
  inappropriate treatment, 175
behavioural services, 204
benzodiazepines, 146, 154
  behavioural problems, 174
Betz cells, 114, 116
bilateral synchrony, secondary, 153
biofeedback techniques, 144
birth
  complications, 3
  see also prematurity
body image, 122–123, 143
  establishment, 146
bone
  age, 142, 146
  deformity management, 106–110
  long bone torsion correction, 103
bone mineral content, 142
botulinum toxin injection, 99, 132
  hamstrings, 104
  muscle tone
    measurement, 134

207

grasp, 121–122
  hand function deficit, 56
  precision, 121
  restoration, 144
  visuomotor skills, 121–122
  voluntary, 128
grasp reflex, 115, 121, 124, *125*
  release, 124
  retained, 127
  voluntary muscle contraction, 128
grip, 122
  opposing pincer, 114
  weak, 128, *129*
growth, 58
  disturbance, 141–142
guilt, 1

H

haemangioma, facial capillary, 155
haemorrhagic infarction, 2
haemosiderosis, cerebral, 163
hallucinations, 171
hallux valgus, 69
hamstrings
  abnormal neurological function, 104
  shift, 105
  spasticity/contracture, 104
    surgical management, 104–105
hand
  anatomy of function, 113–114
  association area, 117
  athetoid movements, 58
  complexity, 113
  coordination, 121
  distal power loss, 132
  dominance in language lateralization, 183
  drop, 55
  early postnatal development, 124
  fisted, 124, 125
  function improvement, 144
  loss of learned skills, 130–132
  manipulation, 122
  neuroanatomy of function, 114–120
  normal maturation of function, 120–122
  regard, 121
  sensory function impairment, 55–56
  sensory loss, 73
  skills, 119
    loss severity, 132
    measurement, 131–132
  speed loss, 132
  splints, 77
head circumference, 58
hearing, 60
helplines, 197
hemianopia, 73

hemidecortication, 163
hemiepilepsy, intractable, 163
  early onset with developmental arrest, 152
  hemispherectomy, 162
Hemi-Help, 195, 196, 203
  needs of membership, 199–200, 201
  organization, 197–199
  services, 199
hemihypoplasia, 72
hemimegalencephaly, 20–21, 163
  seizure outcome, 165
hemiparesis
  MRI-based classification, 37–49
  prevalence, 47
  severity assessment, 164
hemiplegia, postconvulsive chronic, 22, *24*
hemispherectomy, 162–165
  anatomical, 163, 164
  behavioural improvement, 166
  functional, 163, 164
  modified, 163
  Sturge–Weber syndrome, 158
hemispheres
  asymmetry, 20, 21
  maldevelopment, 4
  surgical resection of infarcted region, 144
hemispheric dominance, 118
hemispheric side of injury
  cognitive function reorganization, 187–188
  language skills, 184
  letter knowledge, 187
  reading abilities, 187
  seizures, 184–185
  see also left-hemisphere injury
hemispherotomy, 163
hemisyndrome, 123–124
heredity, 2
heterotopia, 19, 28
hindfoot deformity, 108
hip
  abduction, 89, 92, *93*
  adduction, 67, 68, 89, 92, *93*
  adductor abnormality, 105–106
  coronal plane deviations, 89, *93*
  flexion deformity, 105–106
  increased sagittal-plane motion of the non-involved
    side, 90–91
  reduced range of motion, 86–87, *88*
  rotation, 56, 68, 69–70, 72, 77
    excessive internal, 88
    external, 90, 91, 106–107
homunculus, 117
hydrocephalus, 163
  shunt-treated, 60
hyperactive reflexes, 6
hyperkinetic behaviour, 167–168

hyperkinetic syndrome, 167
hypertonus, 72, 140
   extensor, 124
   measurement, 134
   rigid, 68
   spastic, 67, 76–77
hypoplasia, 70–71
hypotonia, 53–54
   relative, 124
hypoxic–ischaemic lesions, 9, 21–22, *23, 24*

I

Ilizarov device, 109
imaging *see* computerized tomography (CT); magnetic
   resonance imaging (MRI); neuroimaging
inattention, 170
incoordination, 119
infants, 75–77
infection, intrauterine, 14
inheritance, dominant, 3
intellect, 75
interventions, family views, 204
intracranial haemorrhage, 15
   hemiplegic CP, 12
   imaging, 12–13
   perinatal, 11
   preterm babies, 10
intraventricular haemorrhage, periventricular lesions
   with myelin defect, 46
involuntary movement, 119
IQ, 172
   hemisphere injury, 181
   stability, 182
irritability, 170

J

joint range of motion, 69, 145
   measurement, 133
   muscle length, 140
joints
   kinematic plots, 82–83
   passive movement, 141, 145
   sinusoidal flexion/extension, 135

K

kinaesthetic memory, 116, 117, 131
knee
   abnormal neurological function, 104
   excessive flexion, 84, 85, *86*
   flexion deformity, 105
   hyperextension, 56
     in stance, 85–86, *87*
   reduced/delayed peak flexion in swing, 86
knee immobilizer, 98
kyphoscoliosis, 74

L

lamotrigine, 154
language
   function reorganization, 179–180
   lateralization and hand dominance, 183
   neural plasticity, 179–180
   neural systems, 179
language development, 60, 164
   delay/deviance, 171
language skills
   children, 182–185
   cognitive ability, 183
   hemispheric side of injury, 184
   perservation, 181
lateral column shortening, 108
lateralization, 180
   dichotic listening, 183–184
   language, 183
learning difficulties, 185–187
   seizures, 188
learning disability, 59
   cortical–subcortical lesions, 44
   periventricular lesions with myelin defect, 45–46
left-hemisphere injury
   language skills, 184
   letter knowledge, 187
   neuropsychological profile, 189–190
   reading abilities, 187
   seizures, 184–185, 190–191
leg
   flexion, 115
   length discrepancy, 109
   lengthening, 109, 146
   shortening, 58, 71, 72
leptomeningeal angioma, 155
leptomeningeal glioneuronal heterotopia, 19
letter knowledge, 187
leukomalacia, 2
   periventricular, 9, 10, 29, *30*
     risk factors, 14
   subcortical, 31
lever arm disease, 106
lift, 122
limb
   lengthening, 146
   posture, 138–139
   rejection, 143
   see also lower limb; upper limb
linear sebaceous naevus syndrome, 164
lissencephaly, 18–19, 28
listening, dichotic, 183–184, 185
literacy development, 186, 187
locomotor development, 72–73
London Hemiplegia Register (LHR), 195, 196
low birthweight babies, 3, 4
   see also small for gestational age babies

lower limb
  dwarfing, 141–142
  posture, 138–139
  treatment programme, 143
  see also ankle; foot; hip; leg
lower motor neurone impairments, 59
lumbopelvic motion, 110

M

magnetic resonance imaging (MRI), 26, 27
  cerebral malformations, 28, 32
  classification basis, 37–49
    cerebral malformations, 44, *45*
    cortical–subcortical lesions, 42–44
    definitions, 41
    gestational age, 41
    grouping, 38–40, 41–48
    learning disability, 41
    normal MRI findings, 48
    periventricular lesions with myelin defect, 45–47
    periventricular white matter hyperintense lesions, 41–42
    subcortical white matter lesions, 48
    technique, 40
  pathological diagnosis, 205
  Sturge–Weber syndrome, 156, 157
  technique, 34
  use, 33–34
maldevelopment of hemispheres, 4
mana obscena, *127*, 128
management, 74–79
manifestations, early, 53–54
manipulative skill failure, 125
maple syrup urine disease, 20
maternal factors, 3, 4
  predisposing to CP, 14
maternal ill-health, 4
mathematical abilities, 186, 191
metacarpophalangeal joints, *127*, 128
metatarsal osteotomy, multiple, 108
metatarsus adductus, 107–108
microgyria, 155
midfoot, closing-wedge osteotomy, 108
mind-reading skills, 171–172
minicolumns of Mountcastle, 116
mirror dyspraxia, 142
mirror movement, 128
misery, 169
mitochondrial respiratory chain deficiency, 20
Moro reflex, 120–122
motion, resistance to, 134
motor acts, complex, 118
motor association areas, 117
motor cortex, 116–118
  modules, 116
motor disability

leg dominated, 15
  manifestation, 1
motor impairment, 54–57
movement
  clumsiness, 119
  disorder treatment, 76
  full-range passive, 77
  information passage, 118
  involuntary, 119
  resistance to, 133
  speed, 130
  weakness, 127–129, *130*
multihandicap pattern, 61
multiple lower-extremity procedure (MLEP), 101
muscle
  asymmetrical tone, 124
  biomechanical change, 140
  biomechanical resistance, 133
  electrical contraction, 133
  exercise, 144
  growth failure, 145
  lengthening, 140
  plastic change, 145
  release for wrist position, 145
  resistance, 133
  rigidity, 135
  short, 137
  stretch, 135
  stretching, 145
  vibration, 145
muscle spindle, secondary endings, 137
muscle tone, 57, *58*
  abnormalities, 132–133
  measurement, 133–134
  torque generators, 133–134
musculotendinous lengths, 110
myelin defect, 45–47
myoclonic jerks, 150
myoclonus, 152
  negative, 150, 152

N

negativistic behaviour, 169, 170
neonates, diagnosis, 123–124
neural networks, 179
neuroblast migration, 27–28
neurodevelopmental problems, 167
neurodevelopmental treatment, 76
neuroimaging, 26–27
  brain lesions, 8–9, 10, 15
  choice of method, 33–34
  see also computerized tomography (CT); magnetic resonance imaging (MRI)
neurological findings, 57–58
neurological impairment in learning difficulties, 185–186

213